Ana Virgínia De Almeida Figueiredo

Emerging food risks: Regulation, conflicts and tensions

Ana Virgínia De Almeida Figueiredo

Emerging food risks: Regulation, conflicts and tensions

A Brazilian experience

ScienciaScripts

Imprint
Any brand names and product names mentioned in this book are subject to trademark, brand or patent protection and are trademarks or registered trademarks of their respective holders. The use of brand names, product names, common names, trade names, product descriptions etc. even without a particular marking in this work is in no way to be construed to mean that such names may be regarded as unrestricted in respect of trademark and brand protection legislation and could thus be used by anyone.

Cover image: www.ingimage.com

This book is a translation from the original published under ISBN 978-3-330-75623-6.

Publisher:
Sciencia Scripts
is a trademark of
Dodo Books Indian Ocean Ltd. and OmniScriptum S.R.L publishing group

120 High Road, East Finchley, London, N2 9ED, United Kingdom
Str. Armeneasca 28/1, office 1, Chisinau MD-2012, Republic of Moldova, Europe
Printed at: see last page
ISBN: 978-620-6-35872-5

SUMMARY

To Ana Theresa, Joao Carlos and Lucas Freitas, my children, my loves.

ACKNOWLEDGMENTS

Despite the intense and systematic individual effort to complete this thesis, I recognize that it contains a plurality of intellectual supports, emotional influences and shared experiences, stemming from the different interrelationships I have established in the academic and professional environment. For this reason, I would like to start by thanking all those phenomenal individuals I have come across in the course of my history in the field of health surveillance, and who have created opportunities for me to learn and improve myself. The inspiration for the object studied is the result of the restlessness that arose from long debates with these people, all figures in my life.

However, it is necessary to highlight some of these personalities:

- To the mass of Brazilian workers who, in their hard daily work and life, contribute materially to the existence of public universities, despite the fact that a small contingent of them occupy this social space in order to qualify. I hope this thesis is a way of giving them back part of that investment.
- To my advisor, Prof. Dr. Elisabetta Recine, for instructing and guiding me through all the stages of this intellectual construction process, with great competence, patience and affection. A very special thank you to her.
- To my co-supervisor, Prof. Dr. Renata Monteiro, for her valuable contributions, promptness and support throughout my academic activities.
- To Dr. Patrick Dahlet, for the fortuitous and fruitful encounter, as well as for the work with words, which allowed me to unveil the obscure traces of discourses. It was an experience that helped strengthen our affectionate companionship on the winding path of life.
- To the Coordination for the Improvement of Higher Education Personnel - CAPES/Ministry of Education for granting me a doctoral-sandwich scholarship, with which I was able to carry out part of my research at the Universitat Rovira i Virgili, Tarragona-Spain.
- To Dr. Mabel Gracia of the Universitat Rovira i Virgili- Tarragona/Spain for her welcome and contributions to the development of this thesis.
- To the professors and colleagues of the Post-Graduate Program in Human Nutrition for

the different collaborations provided in the vast field of nutrition science.

- To the Health Secretariat of the Federal District, in the person of the Undersecretary for Health Surveillance, Dr. Marilia Cunha, for the institutional support during my academic activity.

- To the Director of the Health Surveillance of the Federal District, Manoel Silva Neto, to the Food Manager, André Godoy Ramos, and to my immediate boss Dillian Adelaine Cesar da Silva for their kindness, understanding and indispensable support in the most intense moments of this work.

- To all the interviewees who kindly gave their valuable time to answer the interview questions and who enriched the content of this thesis.

- To my wonderful friend and work companion, Reginalice Maria da Graça Bueno, with whom I always share the sweet and bitter stories of life. Thank you so much, both for your willingness to help me balance the flavors of events and for your encouragement in my academic adventures.

- To Rosane Maria Franklin Pinto and Elisabete Gonçalves Dutra, colleagues at Anvisa, for their promptness in clarifying my doubts and for carrying out the test interview, which were essential for the preparation of the thesis.

- To my dear work colleagues, Wanusa, Eva, Gisele and Socorro, for their cordial attention and understanding in times of absence.

- To my eternal friends, who reinvigorated Health Surveillance, Joâo Batista de Lima Filho, Silvia Amaral Vignola and Sheila Maria Gomes Castanhola, through whom I learned how to deal with this conflicting field of health work.

- To my adorable children, Ana Theresa and Joâo Carlos, who give me a whirlwind of emotions, but love is the imperative. I'd like to take this opportunity to answer your tireless question: "When will it end, Mom?" It's over.

- To Clàudia Camurça, Joâo's dear aunt, for the care and affection she gave to my son when I was away doing my doctorate.

- To my dear partner, Maria Félix Pereira, for her daily work managing the house and my children, with so much attention, affection and responsibility, which was indispensable in facing this academic challenge.

- To my family, especially Andréa Figueiredo, for the affectionate relationship and mutual commitment. Thank you, my dear sister!

Strange what is not strange. Take the usual as inexplicable. Be perplexed by everyday life. Try to find a remedy for the abuse But don't forget

That abuse is always the rule.

(*The Exception and the Rule, Bertolt Brecht*)

FIGUEIREDO, Ana Virginia, A. University of Brasilia, November 2014. **Emerging food risks: regulation, conflicts and tensions; a Brazilian experience**. Supervisor: Elisabetta Recine. Co-supervisor: Renata Monteiro.

SUMMARY

Over the last few decades, world society and Brazil have been facing emerging food risks, associated with the rapid growth of obesity and other chronic non-communicable diseases (CNCDs). Among the causal factors of these diseases are physical inactivity and the consumption of unhealthy food products, high in fat, sugar and sodium. These products are the result of transformations in the food production and marketing system, fostered by the process of economic globalization, which strives to strengthen the massification of food consumption. This has created an environment that changes lifestyles, daily eating habits and nutritional status. As a result, regulating the nutritional profile of these products is one of the intervention measures recommended by international organizations, to be applied by public control institutions in different countries. The general aim of this study is to analyse the understanding that different subjects, linked to the market, public authorities and organized civil society, have of the transformations and implications of regulation strategies active in the market. This is a qualitative investigation whose aim is to explore the meanings that constitute and construct the reality that permeates emerging food risks and the control of unhealthy food products, based on the theoretical framework of Depth Hermeneutics (THOMPSON, 2000), with the discourses of these subjects as the analytical foundation. Based on the results, it can be said that these risks are a reflection of the dynamics of the global economy, whose regulation takes place in an environment of dispute which, as a rule, does not always favor the interests of collective health. For market players, regulation is an authoritarian and ineffective attitude, with the population being the main culprit for the consequences on their health, by adopting sedentary behavior and excessive food consumption. The alternative is to implement flexible, voluntary measures, such as the agreements the government has established with business entities to gradually reduce nutrient levels; the government would only have to promote food education among the population. For public authorities and civil society, there is recognition of the interconnection between these products and NCDs, which makes most of them defend the practice of regulation. For them, the Agreements are fragile and indicate that the government has acted in a way that seeks the least political damage and economic impact for the market, despite the damage caused to the population. Based on the analysis presented, we conclude that fair regulation requires negotiating clear rules, guided by the principle of promoting and protecting public health, with the participation of the three key subjects identified - public authorities, the market and civil society - and the adoption of conduct that benefits society as a whole, delimiting the rights and duties of each subject that acts in the field of health regulation.

Keywords: Food risks. Health regulation. Health surveillance. Food health control.

PRESENTATION

My first work experience, after completing my Specialization in Public Health and Social Medicine at the Federal University of Paraiba, was joining the technical team of the Ministry of Health's National Food Health Surveillance Division. It was 1985, a time of democratic reconstruction, when public institutes were beginning to rediscuss their purpose and adjust their practices to the New Republic. Unraveling health surveillance was a challenge for me, as it was a subject that had been insufficiently covered during my undergraduate and postgraduate courses. So I took advantage of the rich political and technical context and improved myself during the ongoing process of revitalizing and adjusting institutional practice. There was a real effervescence of change. Everything was being rediscovered and rebuilt in an atmosphere that encouraged dynamism, creativity and participation.

This was my first work experience: health surveillance as part of the scope of public health. From there, I built my professional and academic career. Without losing focus on health surveillance, I had the opportunity to work in two administrative spheres, the federal and the district, as well as in technical support, at the Laboratòrio de Saùde Pública do Distrito Federal, and in an academic institution, the Nùcleo de Estudos em Saùde Pública at the University of Brasilia. This allowed me to explore the different facets and levels of intervention involved in health surveillance and to recognize it as a broad, highly conflictive and increasingly strategic field of action for the protection of collective health.

It was in the 1990s that the concept of health risk was incorporated into the practice of health surveillance and became the central focus of our concern. A risk whose concept insists on being eminently "technical" only hides the "political plot" that runs through the course from the appearance of the risk to decision-making.

So, focusing on the emerging food risks that threaten Brazilian and world society and the actions of the institutes responsible for controlling food risks, I decided to take some time out to explore the technical, political, social and economic complexity surrounding this issue.

The content of this thesis is laid out in six sequential chapters, a conclusion and bibliographical references. The first chapter corresponds to the *Introduction*, which presents a general approach to the impact of food risks on public health, followed by a discussion of the theoretical-methodological framework and details of the steps adopted for the empirical investigation.

In the second chapter, *Food and Health Risks*, a brief overview is given of the social transformations that have led to changes in the cultural conduct of food and that have given dynamism to food risks, as well as exploring the concept of health risk, highlighting its socio-political significance.

The third chapter, *Food Products and Health: a multifaceted analysis*, deals with the actions of supranational agencies in the international regulation of food, the conduct of national institutes aimed at improving the nutritional profile of food and, finally, the globalization of food products, focusing on the characteristics of the products and the artifices used by the market to commercialize them.

The fourth chapter, *The Dynamics of Transitions: dietary, nutritional and epidemiological*, discusses the technical bases of the dietary transition and the nutritional transition and briefly considers the rising prevalence of obesity and other CNCDs in Brazil and around the world, and their respective causal factors.

In the fifth chapter, *Food regulation: the challenge of governing the market*, we look at the basis of the legal provisions for food health surveillance and the transformations of the federal health control body, focusing on its advances and weaknesses, as well as the new modality of action created by the federal government to intervene in the nutritional quality of food products.

The final chapter, *Food Risks and Regulation: visions of social subjects*, discusses the data, consisting of the interpretation of the discourses of the subjects investigated, highlighting the dissonances and obstacles to preventing food risks, the generation and variations of discursive positions on food and nutrition, and the different types of ideology and interests that involve the discourses of the groups of these social subjects.

Finally, the *Conclusion* reinforces the idea that the process of regulating food brings with it a conflict of technical and political interests and, for this reason, there is a need to build it democratically in order to achieve a fair result for society as a whole.

1 INTRODUCTION

1.1 Food risks and their impact on the population's nutritional profile

The theme of this work is anchored in the premise that food is essential to human life, as it is a source of nutrients necessary for growth, development and health. In addition to this vital biological function, food is also one of the most precious forms of cultural expression, forming part of the intangible heritage of different peoples and nations. Thus, it is the fusion of these two components, the biological and the socio-cultural, that makes up the universe of food.

Crises related to the scarcity, contamination, distribution and unequal availability of food are part of human history and have an impact on people's nutritional and health profiles (CHAVES, 1978; FAO, 2009). This has led to systematic imbalances in the quality and/or quantity of food consumed, which generate risks to individual and collective health. At the start of the 21st century, the United Nations Food and Agriculture Organization (FAO) estimates that around 12.5% of the world's population is still undernourished - due to a deficit in energy consumption - and 26% of children are chronically malnourished. These results increase the economic and social costs (higher health care costs, lower productivity at work, etc.) for all countries (FAO, 2013).

When food is consumed in quantities lower than nutritional needs, it is inevitable that disorders will appear which, depending on the intensity and duration of the deficiency, will cause irreversible damage to health, jeopardizing the regular development of life, according to classic nutrition studies (BEATON & McHENRY, 1966; MITCHELL et al, 1978; CHAVES, 1978; TORUN & CHEW; 2003).

Thus, for a long time, the focus of attention given to food was concentrated on studies involving the relationship between insufficient production and consumption and the nutritional deficiencies of populations. These included endemic malnutrition, hypovitaminosis and other types of deficiency, which for decades was the central theme of Nutrition and Public Health. This was the characteristic of nutritional epidemiology[1] until the end of the 1970s: when malnutrition in poor countries took on importance due to its high prevalence and was related to high infant mortality rates (MONTEIRO et al,

1 Nutritional epidemiology is based on the concept that aspects of diet can influence the occurrence ofdiseases in individuals, both diseases originating from insufficient or excessive consumption of dietary factors and those resulting from contamination of food by biological agents, chemicals or natural compounds present in food (WILLET, 1990).

1993; TORUN & CHEW, 2003; POPKIN, 2006; WHO, 1990).

With the progress made in food science and technology, which began in the 1940s (FAO; WHO, 2006), and which led to improvements in food processing and preservation systems, especially advances in additive chemistry (PHILIPPI, 2000), it became possible to expand food trade at local and international level, especially in processed products. As a result of the intense circulation of food between countries, other forms of transnational health risk have also emerged. Thus, food is beginning to be approached by supranational organizations (FAO & WHO, 2006) based on its paradoxical nature, expressed by its ability to provide nutrients to promote health and, at the same time, to harbor contaminants capable of spreading disease.

As a consequence of this commercial exchange of foodstuffs, in the 1960s the issue of "food" was progressively placed on the agenda of international and strategic interests with a view to standardization, due to the potential threats posed by the spread of diseases caused by contaminants. This broadened the range of concerns about food, since the issues linked to the binomial of food shortages and malnutrition that had already surrounded them still persisted.

In order to contain any events that might hinder trade relations and the preservation of people's health, multilateral organizations such as the United Nations Food and Agriculture Organization (FAO) and the World Health Organization (WHO) took on the responsibility of regulating aspects that could guarantee the health of food traded between countries. The measure adopted was the establishment of international health recommendations to control biological and chemical agents resulting from practices related to agricultural and industrial activities. Thus, the FAO/WHO *Codex Alimentarius* Commission2 was responsible for developing the food standards program, aimed at protecting consumer health and ensuring fair practices in food trade (FAO/WHO, 2005).

Despite the persistence of nutritional deficiencies and the challenges of autonomy in food production and distribution that many peoples face (WHO, 2010; WHO, 2011), the last two decades have seen the coexistence of two major risks to the health of the world's population related to food consumption. Both condense a set of common characteristics that can be summarized as follows: they expose all individuals to harm, although the socially vulnerable are the most affected; they transcend continents; they can be easily controlled and, finally, they are related to the transformations in the economic logic of food production that arise and expand as a result of globalization (WHO, 2002a; WHO;

2008).

Globalization is a complex and multifaceted process that encompasses economic, political and social issues. With the globalization of markets, through the expansion and intensification of capitalist production relations, under the support of new technologies, the recreation of the international division of labour and product innovation (IANNI, 2007), a type of consumer society is being consolidated (BAUMAN, 1999). This leads to the strengthening of transnational actors, especially corporations ([2]), which interfere with the sovereignty, identity and power of national states (BECK, 1999).

As far as health risks are concerned, the first group, which has become more complex over the decades, refers to outbreaks of food-borne diseases[3] (FBD), with transnational coverage, rapid spread and frequent occurrence, caused by common agents and emerging pathogens (ALTEKRUSE; SWERDLOW, 1996; KATZ et al, 1999; WHO; 2008) or from air, water and soil pollution and other chemical agents that appear at different points in the production chain (WHO, 2003a). The risks of contamination by agents with antimicrobial resistance that compromise the efficiency of conventional control measures should also be highlighted in this group (KAFERSTEIN et al, 1997; TRAUXE, 1997; TAORMINA; BEUCHAT; SLUTSKER, 1999).

With regard to the second group, which are considered emerging risks linked to food and which have reached a global scale over the last few decades, we highlight the risk of obesity[4] and other related chronic non-communicable diseases (NCDs), the expansion of which covers all continents (WHO, 2004a). Obesity, recognized today for its pandemic nature, is mainly the result of behavioral, social, environmental and economic changes, which have intensified the imbalance between energy consumption and expenditure, and is closely associated with the current characteristics of the food consumed, which has a high energy density (MONTEIRO, 2009; MONTEIRO, 2010; WHO, 2004a).

Advances in food technology, coupled with the support of the regulatory apparatus, have both enabled the formulation of relatively safe products in microbiological terms, and the creation of poor or unhealthy products in nutritional terms. These are products with a

---

2 This Commission was created in 1961 by the FAO and WHO, with the aim of developing an international food code, emphasizing safety and quality aspects, to protect consumer health and discipline the food trade.
3 Based on the World Health Organization's definition, "*foodborne* diseases" consist of diseases commonly transmitted by food and comprise a wide range of signs and symptoms caused by pathogenic microorganisms, parasites, chemical contaminants and biotoxins (WHO, 2007).
4 In this study, "overweight" is the general term used to refer to overweight and obesity together. Whether the terms - overweight, obesity or overweight - are mentioned independently or in isolation will depend on the study being referred to.

high energy density, high saturated fat, salt and free sugar content and low in essential nutrients, which are made available on the market at affordable prices and therefore stimulate consumption[5] (WHO, 2003b; WHO 2006). Furthermore, these products have had a negative impact on people's traditional eating habits, making it difficult to practise a healthy diet (POPKIN, 2006).

As described above, these food products are responsible for emerging food risks. Risks defined by the potential of these products to cause harm to human health, due to certain types of excess nutrients - hazards - present in their composition, which is defined from formulas based on processed and low-nutrient ingredients. Thus, it is the systematic consumption of these food products by the population that has a negative impact on food and nutrition. This is the context in which the obesity pandemic is emerging and other NCDs are developing.

According to the WHO, the prevalence of obesity on the European continent fluctuated between 5% and 23% in men and between 7% and 36% in women between 1999 and 2004 (WHO, 2006). However, in previous periods, from 1988 to 1994, it had already reached the American adult population, aged between 20 and 74, at levels of 19.9% to 24.9% for men and women respectively (WHO, 2004a). In Brazil, the most recent data on the nutritional status of the Brazilian population reveals that the age groups of 10 to 19 years and 20 years and over have prevalences of obesity of 4% and 14.8%; for overweight, the figures correspond to 19.4% and 49% respectively (BRASIL/IBGE, 2010). The evolution of obesity in adults in Brazil has been taking place over the last 25 years, and has been observed in the Northeast and Southeast regions of the country (BATISTA FILHO; RISIN, 2003).

Generally speaking, this reconfiguration of the population's nutritional profile stems from a multiplicity of factors involving changes in the social environment, the expansion of global trade in food products without appropriate sanitary control, alterations in food consumption patterns, the introduction of new food production processes and increased human interference in native environments (NEWELL et al, 2010; ALTEKRUSE; SWERDLOW,1996; KAFERSTEIN; MONTARJEMI; BETTCHER, 1997; WHO, 2008). In addition, it has been favored by an increase in the consumption of fat and sugar added to diets, thanks to the sharp rise in the availability of animal products and other

5 These foods also include energy-dense drinks. They can also be referred to by other names such as: unhealthy foods or food products, nutritionally inadequate foods, foods or products that pose a high risk to health and ultra-processed foods.

industrialized products, as opposed to the low consumption of foods rich in fiber and whole grains (POPKIN, 2001) and foods from the traditional diet (WHO, 2004a).

Undoubtedly, obesity and food-borne diseases are part of the global panorama of diseases of relevance to public health, which can be perfectly considered as one of the types of supranational risks, due to their breadth and effects, reaching as mentioned by Giddens (2008). For the author, these are forms of risk with intercontinental reach and undetermined effects, which continually arise and are renewed as a consequence of contemporary social processes. Although the harmful impacts are extensive, the most socially vulnerable population groups in the countries are the most affected.

The availability and systematic stimuli for the consumption of globally circulated food products, which are high in calories, low in nutrients and have attributes of practicality, induce the population to give preference to such products and, consequently, expose them to the risk of contracting these diseases.

Addressing the risks of food today forces us to immerse ourselves in a scenario led by the market, which enjoys the effervescent dynamism of production technologies, the continuous creation of goods and inputs, as well as the improvement of commercial strategies to stimulate consumption. At the other end of the spectrum are consumer-citizens stunned by the excessive diversity of food products available to them and uninformed about the harmful effects these products can have on their health. Both stakeholders suffer from the controlling influence of government institutes, whose action is limited. This results in a mismatch between the rapid pace of outbreaks of food-borne health phenomena and the reduced political and operational capacity to satisfactorily control health risks.

It should also be pointed out that the advent of the obesity pandemic and the increase in NCDs require a new look at food-related health risks, demanding reflections and changes in the traditional way of conceiving the object of "health surveillance" in the field of food and exercising regulation over it. Health surveillance is understood here as [...] *a set of actions capable of eliminating, reducing or preventing health risks and intervening in health problems arising from the environment, the production and circulation of goods and the provision of services of interest to health* (BRASIL; CONASS, 2003a). These actions are carried out in a decentralized manner by the three levels of the Unified Health System.

This scenario - with a new socially generated risk - is in place and it weakens the health of the population, challenges official control institutes and prompts us to raise the following hypothesis: despite recognizing that public regulation of food is one of the political-operational strategies needed to intervene in emerging food risks, the political forces in the current state are insufficient to effectively implement it, due to the power of the industries - which react by attributing responsibility for nutritional disorders to consumers and minimizing the demands of civil society.

Considering the aforementioned assumptions, managing food risks from a health and nutritional perspective requires, at the very least, adjustments within regulatory bodies and food-producing industries, to incorporate concerns about curbing obesity and its comorbidities. Of course, it also means broadening the range of possibilities for public intervention in the health problems prevalent in the population.

This expansion will (could) lead to a restrictive or limiting aspect of the freedom of industrial production. Regulatory institutes will have to strengthen their technical and political back-up to enable them to dialog with strategic subjects and manage the conflicting interests that permeate activities of this nature.

In the current logic of how society works, emerging food risks, related to obesity and other CNCDs, behave like continually growing threats, requiring control. But this measure runs counter to proposals that advocate reducing the functions of the state, justified by the self-sufficiency of the market in managing its business. In these cases, as some authors advocate, risks are the driving force behind the improvement of regulatory activities, since it is necessary to contain the uncertainties and insecurities derived from modern technology and science, used in the manufacture of products, goods and services made available to society (LUCCHESE, 2003; BODSTEIN, 2000).

It should be noted that health regulation must follow different guidelines to those applied to market regulation in general. Regulation in the field of health is a process of risk management of potential deficiencies or adversities that may arise from the consumption or use of products of interest to health and affect the community (CARVALHEIRO, 2001; LUCCHESE, 2008). From this point of view, the primary purpose of regulation is to be a vehicle for public health policies. It should be emphasized that the nature of this state activity is not confined exclusively to the drafting of rules (OLIVEIRA; ELIAS, 2012), but involves other various forms of action.

In the health sector, state intervention in the conduct of the productive sector is imperative in order to guarantee the defense and protection of public health when there are situations involving risks; a legitimate procedure provided for in Brazilian legal provisions (BRASIL; CONASS 2003a, 2003b; 2003c).

In the field of health surveillance, regulation, as an intervention in risk, always presupposes the combination of multidisciplinary technical knowledge and political positioning, and has several components that go beyond the state's private inspection of objects of interest to health itself. Health regulation, one of the components of risk analysis[6] (risk management), includes measures such as regulation, investigation, inspection, monitoring, control, auditing and evaluation, which are adopted by the state in order to contain the risk object or event that threatens the health of the population (CARVALHEIRO, 2001; LUCCHESE, 2008).

Currently, Brazilian health regulation is developing from a process of collective construction, with the active involvement of different subjects, including, in one of its phases, space for the participation of the population in general. Representatives of the market[7] , organized civil society, universities and related public health institutions are part of this process. It is in this environment that scientific knowledge, political and ideological positions, expectations and strategic guidelines for protecting the population from food risks come together. It is under these different perspectives - market, public authorities and civil society - interspersed with conflicts of interest, that the possible consensus to make it possible to control the risks of the nutritional components of food is gradually modulated.

Although formally democratic, these regulatory decisions still need to be adjusted to the bilateral and multilateral agreements signed, as in the case of the Southern Common Market-Mercosur and the World Trade Organization-WTO, and to international standards, such as those established by the FAO/WHO *Codex Alimentarius*. In certain circumstances, these processes act as a brake on the progress of proposals that are closer to the interests of collective health. However, the sanitary regulation practiced in the daily life of the control institutes is still the only effective state intervention measure in the interest of collective health, and it is relatively democratic. Used to adjust market

---

6 According to FAO/WHO (2005), risk analysis is a process that consists of three components: risk assessment, risk management and risk communication. Assessment is a process based on technical-scientific knowledge, which serves to guide risk management - when the different options for intervention are evaluated, in consultation with interested parties, with reference to the protection of consumer health and the promotion of fair trade practices.

7The food market is an expression used in a broad sense, referring to all the commercial operations established in the different stages of the food production system that are aimed at human consumption. It also encompasses all the members of the food production system, in its different stages, which can be referred to in this study as productive sectors, regulated sectors or economic sectors.

practices, this is the way to demand the adoption of measures to prevent and control the risks of products and services offered to society, as well as to apply sanctions and penalties when there is non-compliance or deviation from the defined rules.

The main object of this study is to elucidate the points of convergence and divergence, the arguments for regulation, the commitments to public health and the limits of political action that arise when this issue is put on the agenda.

In this sense, investigating the discourse of the subjects involved in this agenda - representatives of public authorities, the market, organized civil society and an international body - will make it possible to elucidate the significant motivations that guide their actions around the problematic of this study. At the same time, we hope to obtain answers to the following questions: What are the risks of food, recognized by these subjects, that can lead society to develop chronic diseases? What are the political-institutional strategies and conflicts faced by different subjects to contain emerging food risks? How is the regulation of the nutritional components of food accepted in order to contain the advance of obesity and other CNCDs? Is there a shared commitment on the part of the subjects to make the control of the nutritional components of food an institutional practice?

Based on these considerations, the following objectives were formulated for this study:

a) *General Objective*: To analyze the understanding of the different subjects involved in the food and nutrition agenda about emerging food risks, and the public regulatory action involved, in order to contribute to its improvement.

b) *Specific Objectives*:

- Identify the meanings attributed to emerging food risks and their relationship with the expansion of the global food market;

- To characterize the construction of meanings about the conduct and regulatory measures adopted by the public authorities to interfere in the quality of food products, due to the evolution of obesity and other NCDs;

- To characterize, in the discourses expressed, the interests that permeate the issue of public action to regulate the nutritional components of food products, as a strategy to intervene in emerging food risks;

- To delineate, based on the statements extracted from the speeches, the responsibilities that each of the subjects attributes to themselves and others, with regard to the prevention and control of emerging food risks.

1.2 Methodological paths of research

Theoretical-methodological framework

The apparently paradoxical relationship between food and health that prevails in contemporary society has stimulated the production of research interested in elucidating the conceptions of individuals and the conduct of institutions on issues of nutrition, as well as risk, regulation and food safety. These topics seem to be progressively gaining ground in local and international scientific literature. In this sense, several studies, from different perspectives, use discursive material, constructed from the subjects' accounts, to evaluate, among other aspects, the consumption of advertising messages on nutrition and the prevention of chronic diseases (HENDERSON et al, 2010), the discourses and beliefs related to food risks (LUPTON, 2005), consumers' perceptions of the traditional and current risks attributed to food (BUCHLER; SMITH; LAWRENCE, 2010) and the conflict that permeates consumption practices, desire *versus* control, with a view to reducing food risks (HALKIER, 2001).

However, it is also not uncommon for these studies to use interviews with representatives of organizations as a source, when the line of research aims to find out the institutional position regarding risk control. Studies of this nature have been carried out on the monitoring of fluoride concentrations in food products (BARDAL et al, 2012), the implementation of the food risk analysis tool (FIGUEIREDO; MIRANDA, 2011) and the analysis of the meanings of health safety (BARBOSA; COSTA, 2010).

Using a primary source of similar data, the object of this study is to understand the relationship between emerging food risks and the view of public regulation expressed by different subjects, based on the assumption that, through the use of language, the meanings that constitute and construct this specific reality can be explored.

The organized representations - of the market[8], of public authorities and of society - make up the main subjects that are relevant to this study. Each of the subjects illustrates a differentiated position in the set of representations, which translates into dominance and confrontation with the object of discussion and their ability to use various pressure mechanisms to adjust it to the interests of the sector they defend. So it is this relationship, involving the object and the subjects mentioned above, that leads us to choose a method

8 In this study, the analytical category "market" refers to the representatives of the production system, especially in the stages that comprise the industrialization and distribution of food products.

capable of providing answers to the following questions: How is the relationship between the nutritional profile of food products and obesity and NCDs, which have been on the rise in Brazilian society over the last decade, understood? What meaning is given to regulating the nutritional profile of food products in order to meet current health needs?

In order to access the subjectivity that permeates the universe of these issues, the Hermeneutics of Depth - HP (THOMPSON, 2000) was chosen as a theoretical and methodological reference to deal with the meanings mobilized by the Symbolic Forms - SF, understanding them as artifices not only of meaning, but also of domination in the social whole. The author conceptualizes SFs (actions, speeches, texts) as significant phenomena interpreted and understood by producer-receiver subjects.

HP allows for the insertion of different types of analysis that deal with the structural characteristics of the FS or the socio-historical conditions of action and interaction, because, according to Thompson (2000), it is an aid to the process of interpretation, in a legitimate and collaborative way. This flexibility of HP allowed for the insertion of the method of Discourse Analysis - DA (ORLANDI, 2010), which will be used at specific moments during the journey that leads to reinterpretation.

According to this author, the field-object and the field-subject form a synthesis. The object under observation and explanation is constructed, in part, by the subjects endowed with understanding, reflection and action, including the potential to trigger a process of transformation of the subject-object field (THOMPSON, 2000).

It should be noted that the effects of the modernization of society, which expand and sophisticate the mechanisms of interaction, have not left the FS immune and have modified its original character. As society has evolved, they have ceased to be the result of exclusively face-to-face interaction, mainly as a result of the development of institutions and the mass media, as well as incorporating economic value into symbolic value[9] , becoming instruments for commercial transactions (THOMPSON, 2000).

In order to analyze the FS as ideological, the author focuses on the study of ideology in complex societies, discarding the idea that its role lies in acting as an inducer of social stability or as an agglutinator of divergent collective interests. Social cohesion is a circumstantial characteristic, which is possibly sustained by the influence of certain factors such as: differentiated values and beliefs, a multiplicity of internal groups *and the*

9 Thompson (2000) states that the economic valuation of symbolic forms is a special condition and stems from the exchange of the symbolic good, carried out in the context of the market.

lack of consensus on a specific issue which makes political action unfeasible. Ideology is based on the interrelationship between meaning and power, and its character is to create and constitute social life, through the dynamism of the circulation of actions and interactions, in which FS exchanges take part. These arguments justify our interest in investigating the social uses of PS, as ideological manifestations, inserted in a specific socio-historical context, which take place both in everyday life and in the sphere of institutions, both treated from the conceptual approach of ideology (THOMPSON, 2000).

Having made the above points, the process of signification begins with an exploration of the transcribed texts of the interviews conducted with 13 subjects (representatives of public power, the market and organized civil society), which illustrates the universe of common sense and then continues, as Orlandi (2010) proposes, until the political-ideological commitments mediated by the subjects' language and materialized in discourse are revealed.

Common sense information makes it possible to understand how the intersubjective world, constructed in an environment of sharing and communication, acquires meaning for individuals, allowing them to explain how it works and its internal disorders and to give it objectivity, which is always provisional, due to the dialectical relationship between them and the social world (BERGER; LUCKMANN, 2009). For the authors, language, as a collection of socially produced knowledge, is one of the systems that has the capacity to transcend, connect different facets of everyday life and integrate them into a totality endowed with meaning, which forms the common sense of reality - an image that is apparently clear when people read it, but which is essentially obscure when analyzed.

This is because the symbolic object is impregnated with the binomial of desire and power, which is gradually unveiled and decoded through the construction of discourse (FOUCAULT, 1999). The power referred to here by the author is that which passes through the subjects and takes effect in the multiple relationships established in the social world, completely distancing itself from the type instituted from the formal hierarchical structure. Subjects are, at the same time, active receivers and transmitters of power, an act that takes shape through the constitution, reformulation and dissemination of discourses in the dynamics of social interactions. However, if articulated with knowledge, power becomes more cunning, as it is covered with the mask of subtlety and radiates itself in the daily life of human existence without being easily revealed (FOUCAULT, 1982).

In this way, Bourdieu (2009) recognizes that cultural capital (symbolic power) together with economic capital (material power) comprise the two principles of differentiation that can be used in a stratified society to shape the marks of distinction of social groups established within and outside groups. The groups defined on the basis of the composition of capital distinguish themselves in terms of their interests and the positions they take up in society. These differences become relations of force for imposing representations of this space and for taking up positions in the daily struggles aimed at transforming or maintaining it.

In this sense, the subjects investigated here, individuals who carry this double attribute of power-knowledge and who represent technical-political institutions, probably use the technical-scientific basis in their speeches to express the political-ideological interests that will later be identified in their speeches.

When referring to subjects, Thompson (2000) makes two important points. The first is the recognition of the active and therefore critical receiver. The appropriation of the messages received is a process of self-formation and self-understanding, which requires a continuous effort on the part of the individual to understand and make sense of them, contest them and share them. The second consideration points to the historicity of subjects, active human beings who participate in the social world, embedded in historical traditions, the nature of which partly involves a complex cast of meanings and values that are passed down from generation to generation.

In this context, the oral or written word is one of the forms of symbolic manifestation that leads to an understanding of events. However, it is necessary to overcome the condition of opacity and illuminate one of the gestures of meaning present in it (ORLANDI, 2010). For this reason, the art of interpreting words in the form of discourses will be used as a complementary methodological strategy. According to this author, interpreting is the act of abstracting the implicit economy of the discourse from the subjects' speech: the hidden, non-verbalized elements, surrounded by historicity, which translate their political-ideological affiliation and give them meaning and thus transform man and the social environment.

It is then a question of delving into the implicit, the core of discourse, the part that is so secret, inaccessible in all its dimensions, the "never-said" that bears the marks of historical determination (FOUCAULT, 2008). This has repercussions both on the authorship of the speaking subject, since its function is to give unity, meaning and coherence to the discursive object, and on the interpretation of the discursive object, making it an open range of interpretations.

In Thompson's (2000) theoretical framework, the hermeneutics of everyday life is the starting point. The author refers to this preliminary moment as the interpretation of Doxa, that is, the opinions, beliefs and understandings that are held and shared by people in the social world. From this substratum, the subsequent dimensions are explored in order to encompass the totality of the aspects that involve the FS. In this way, and considering that SW is structured and embedded in socio-historical conditions, the framework comprises three analytically distinct dimensions of a complex interpretative process:

- 1- Dimension - Socio-historical analysis - reconstruction of the socio-historical conditions of production, circulation and reception of the PS. It consists of four elements: *space-time situations* (reconstruction of the production and reception environments of the FS); *fields of interaction* (analysis of resources, rules, conventions and social relations); *social institutions* (reconstruction of the relatively stable sets of rules and resources and social relations); and social *structure* (analysis of the relatively stable asymmetries and differences that characterize social institutes and fields of interaction).
- 2≡ dimension - Formal or discursive analysis - provides the basis for a type of analysis focused on the internal organization of the FS (structural characteristics, patterns and relationships), and different types of analysis can be used. In this study, in particular, Discourse Analysis (DA) will be used.

In order to encompass the language-discourse-ideology triad, AD seeks to make speech concrete, making a reflexive journey from description to interpretation. It encompasses new reading gestures, which culminate in the deconstruction of the utterance, by crossing the historical with the linguistic, which enters the sphere of its apparent superficiality, to rescue the materiality of the meaning that is the discourse itself (PECHEUX, 2008).

According to Orlandi (2010), AD makes use of two devices at different moments in the analysis:

a) Theoretical device of interpretation: the one that mediates the movement between description and interpretation. This means making explicit the processes of meaning present in the text and identifying the "unspoken" meanings, understanding how they are constituted;

b) Analytical device: the one constructed by the analyst, based on the nature of the materials analyzed, the question asked, the purpose of the analysis and the different theories that make up the different disciplinary fields (ORLANDI, 2010).

- 3≡ dimension - Interpretation (or reinterpretation). It analyzes the creative construction of possible meanings of what is said, by synthesizing the previous dimensions, highlighting its ideological character, which means (...) *making explicit the connection between the meaning mobilized by the FS and the relations of domination that this meaning maintains* (THOMPSON, 2000).

Field research

This is a qualitative empirical investigation, appropriate for investigating complex social phenomena in the contemporary world (MINAYO, 2006), in which two specific techniques were applied: document analysis and interviews with subjects, both related to the institutions of interest to the research and involving the theme of food risks, regulation, food control, obesity and/or NCDs. The documents refer to institutional materials in the public domain and were analyzed from the perspective of contextualizing the information. As these documents represent one of the constructed versions of the reality observed, there are limitations in using them to validate the statements obtained in interviews (FLICK, 2009).

As for the interviews, the aim was to explore the ideas and meanings that the subjects attributed to the object under investigation. It should be noted that part of the group of subjects is very close to this subject, as it coincides with their daily work activity. Strategic subjects were identified, i.e. those with decision-making power and who participate directly in and/or follow discussions at national and international level on food risks, regulation and control and/or the prevalence of obesity and NCDs in the population.

In view of this, two groups of analysis were formed: *Study of official documents*, which contains the specifications and analysis process of the selected documents, and *Interviews with the subjects*, which mentions the public and private institutions and organized civil society entities that took part in the research, as well as the data collection process.

The procedures for carrying out this research are in accordance with the guidelines and norms that regulate research involving human beings, set out in Resolution No. 196 of October 10, 1996 of the National Health Council. The field research was approved by the Ethics Committee of the Faculty of Health Sciences - UNB, according to Opinion No.° 117/2012.

Study of official documents

The official documents selected and in the public domain include the following: ministerial ordinances, technical reports, terms of commitment, minutes, agreements and draft laws. These documents, with the exception of the draft laws, refer to the years 2007 and 2014 and deal with some of these topics: food, obesity, NCDs, risk and/or regulation. These documents were analyzed considering the purposes of public health and nutrition policy and the current epidemiological-nutritional framework.

In addition, the official website of the Chamber of Deputies of the National Congress was searched for all available bills on the above-mentioned topics, covering the period from 01/01/2000 to 31/12/2013. The cut-off point for the survey of institutional publications was the year 2000, as this was the year the obesity pandemic was officially announced by international organizations. The following keywords were used to search for bills on this site: regulation & food; control & food; advertising & food; and obesity. This collection coincided with the period during which the interviews were conducted.

The institutional documents of the Ministry of Health, the National Health Surveillance Agency and the Chamber of Deputies used are partly described in Chapter IV, or referenced in the bibliography of this work.

Interviews with the subjects

The group of interviewees was made up of 13 subjects representing 12 institutions. According to the type of institution they belonged to, the subjects fell into four categories:

- *institutions of public power*: include five institutions with the power to approve and/or assist in the construction of legal instruments (laws, decrees or regulations) and technical instruments (food monitoring programs, technical guidelines on food, etc.) related to food risk control - the National Health Surveillance Agency - Anvisa/MS, the General Coordination of Food and Nutrition - CGAN/MS, the Ministry of Agriculture, Livestock and Food Supply - MAPA, the Chamber of Deputies of the National Congress and the Federal Council of Nutritionists - CFN.
- *Private market institutions*: These are three national institutions that represent the food industry and regularly participate in the national food regulation process, coordinated by Anvisa/MS and/or MAPA. They are Brazilian Association of Food Industries - ABIA, Brazilian Association of Dietetic Food Industries - ABIAD and Brazilian Association of Pasta and Industrialized Bread & Cake Industries - ABIMA.
- *Civil society institutions:* There are three institutions that participate in the social

control of health and food actions - the National Health Council (CNS), the National Council for Food and Nutritional Security (Consea) and the Institute for Consumer Protection (Idec).

- *International organization:* Pan American Health Organization - PAHO, which works to encourage member countries to improve their health actions, following the guidelines of the World Health Organization - WHO, including in relation to food control and excess weight.

The only public institution in which two subjects were selected for interviews was the Chamber of Deputies. Two parliamentarians were interviewed because of their work on "food and nutrition security" and "food advertising".

In order to carry out the interviews, most of the institutions required contact with a "*gatekeeper*", who is a professional with a previously established relationship with the researcher or indicated by a person known to her, in order to facilitate access to the institution (CRESWELL, 2010). This "gatekeeper" was fundamental in helping to bring the interviewees closer to the researcher, since they are people in strategic hierarchical positions, with complex demands and limited time available.

Prior contact was made with the subjects to provide information about the study and check their acceptance. Initially, two more interviews were planned with the Brazilian Association for the Study of Obesity and Metabolic Syndromes (ABESO) and the Food and Agriculture Organization of the United Nations (FAO), the former being a civil society organization and the latter an international organization. However, due to the lack of confirmation that the interview had been scheduled or the availability of times that didn't coincide with other interviews, the situations were treated as an implicit denial and impossibility, respectively. In cases of agreement, an institutional document was sent by e-mail informing the subjects of the purpose of the research and the relevance of the data to be provided by the representatives of the institutions. The interviewees were then scheduled according to their availability. At the same time, they were sent an invitation letter containing information about the research and the basic precepts relating to research ethics. In order to carry out a total of thirteen interviews, it was necessary to send more than a hundred e-mails and make numerous telephone contacts.

The location of the interview depended on where the interviewee indicated, and almost all of them were interviewed in their own work environment. Before starting the interviews, the interviewees were informed about the purpose of the study, the recording, the confidentiality of the information, the use of the data for academic purposes, the anonymity of the interviewees and then the procedures for reading and signing the Informed Consent Form were carried out, as determined by the Ethics Committee of the University of Brasilia.

The interview was interpersonal and one-to-one, using a semi-structured script and a digital voice recorder, and lasted approximately one hour. The interview script consisted of a single model, so that the interviewees' speeches on the different aspects of the topic under investigation could be compared. The open-ended questions were drawn up with reference to the objectives and research questions, in order to reduce the possibility of deviating from the focus of the research (Chart 1). This type of question allows the subjects to address what they consider to be the most important aspects of the topic with a certain degree of freedom.

TABLE 1: Comparative table of interview questions, objectives and questions.

Questions	Objectives	Interview questions
What are the food risks recognized by these subjects that could lead society to develop chronic diseases?	***General*** Analyze the understanding of the different subjects involved in the food and nutrition agenda. nutrition on emerging food risks and the public regulatory action involved, with a view to contributing to their improvement.	*1 In your opinion, what is the relationship between food and health?* *2How has the consumption of industrialized food affected modern life?* *3What food-related health problems do you currently know about? How can they be avoided?* *4What measures can the government take to prevent food-related illnesses? What about the overweight population?* *5How can health surveillance act on industrialized foods for*
	Specifics Identify the meanings attributed to emerging food risks and their relationship with the expansion of the global food market.	

		the health of the population?
How is it accepted to regulate the nutritional components of food in order to curb the spread of obesity and other CNCDs? **What are the political-institutional strategies underway and the conflicts faced by different subjects in order to contain emerging food risks?**	To characterize the construction of meanings about the conduct and regulatory measures adopted by the public authorities to interfere in food products, due to the evolution of obesity and other CNCDs. Characterize, in the discourses expressed, the interests that permeate the issue of public action to regulate the nutritional components of food products, as a strategy to intervene in food risks.	*6.What is your assessment of the strategy for regulating the nutritional components of processed foods? health surveillance?*
Is there a shared commitment on the part of the subjects to make the control of the nutritional components of food an institutional practice?	To delineate, based on the statements extracted from the speeches, the responsibilities that each of the subjects attributes to themselves and others with regard to the prevention and control of emerging food risks.	*7.What would be the responsibilities of the government and other sectors involved in the process of regulating emerging food risks in order to control overweight? What about your sector?*

The interview protocol was made up of three parts: the first, containing the interviewee's identification data (name of interviewee, location, date, e-mail); the second part, containing the introductory questions for the researcher to get to know the interviewee; and the third, containing the script questions, with a space for recording the information (Appendix 1). Before the fieldwork began, a pre-test was carried out with three subjects from the institutions involved, in order to adjust the script, which resulted in the questions being improved, the sequence of questions being redefined, among other aspects.

The interviews were essential sources of information for this study and were carried out between 26/02/2013 and 06/06/2013 in the cities of São Paulo and Brasilia.

The entire recording was transcribed by the researcher herself as the interviews took place. The recordings were digitized in MP3 format and then checked by the researcher herself. The interviewees were identified in the transcriptions by their first and last names and the acronym of the institution, and were anonymized in the final text and referred to by code.

The codes were made up of letters and numbers. Interviewees from the market, public authorities and civil society had their code start with the letter "M", "p" and "S" respectively, followed by a specific number for each interviewee in the group in question, in sequential order coinciding with the time the interview took place.

A Research Diary was set up to record all the information, comments, ideas and perceptions about the study in progress, as well as the activities carried out in the daily routine of the research, which were used in the preparation of the final draft.

Data analysis plan

The plan for analyzing the interviews was developed using an adaptation of the proposals structured by Orlandi (2010) and Minayo (2006) and consisted of three distinct moments:

a) *Configuration of the corpus*: After an exhaustive reading of the material collected (the transcribed interviews), the text was cut out and grouped into four generic themes, taking into account the objectives of the thesis and the interview script, namely: the interrelationship between food and health in today's life; agreement and regulation; multisectoral action by the government and the subjects' commitments to the issue. Next, the relevant excerpts from the transcripts were organized according to these four generic themes and according to the institutional spaces in which they take place: public authorities, the market, organized civil society and international organizations. From the specific analysis of each theme, the object discourse was constructed.

b) *Discourse-object*: By postulating that discourse objects are progressively constructed, negotiated and enriched by the discursive activity itself, this material was structured as a discourse-object and support for analysis, based on matrix statements considered to be transversal to the set of transcriptions. These matrix statements were extracted from the recurrences of ideas identified in the transcribed texts, observing the characteristics in terms of similarities or divergences, conflicts and contradictions in the arguments used to construct the meanings.

c) *Discourse*: Through the use of the theoretical framework, the elaboration of these extracted matrix statements formed the basis for the analytical reconstruction of the discourses and the explication of the subjects' political-ideological interests in relation to the central issues of this study: food risks and regulation.

Once the discourses had been concluded, a moment of synthesis between the empirical data and the theory, they were integrated into a socio-historical analysis in order to complete the theoretical model proposed by Thompson (2000) and clarify the object under analysis in its complexity, in other words, to reinterpret it.

In order to synthetically represent the multiplicity of discourses around the semantic field in question, we used the model of the Semiotic Square, proposed by Greimas (1970) and presented by Barros (2005), which consists of a visual representation of the logical articulation of the elementary structures extracted from the texts and which underpin the generative path of the discourse. A semiotic square, it is constructed from the relationship between two terms, marked by opposition or difference, and their contradictions. These four terms, situated in four different positions, form relationships between them of contrast (horizontal axis), complementarity (vertical axis) and contradiction (crosses) (BARROS, 2005).

2 FOOD AND HEALTH RISKS

2.1 The contemporary diner: from food to food product

Food for individuals goes beyond a simple act of survival instinct. It condenses a complex set of symbolic and material meanings, typical of human nature, which simultaneously articulates three conditions: it responds to biological need, expresses cultural behavior and represents interaction in a social environment. It is a phenomenon that combines the biological and social reproduction of human groups and is surrounded by a repertoire of representations, beliefs and habits that make up the cultural universe (CONTRERAS; GRACIA, 2011).

In this context, human food is the meeting of nature and culture (MACIEL, 2005). The ritual of food choices, habits and practices derives from collectively constructed knowledge, accumulated and passed down from generation to generation, but not completely inert to the effects of social dynamics. This cultural particularity of food, which is not detached from its origins and is reproduced throughout social life, makes it a historical category (SANTOS, 2005).

Thus, linked to individuals or groups, food tradition remains beyond spaces or social transformations, in other words, it transcends the physical or temporal distance relative to the typical environment in which it circulates, even though it is adaptable to new forms, flavors and food practices. This persistent cultural mosaic constitutes a reference of high symbolic value that refers to origin and taste memory and becomes part of identity (PONS, 2005).

As for the identity relationship with food, Pons (2005) states that it has a double biocultural dimension, both "(...) *as a taste complex shared by a group, and as an internalized symbolic universe that informs those who share it of the boundaries between culture and nature, between what is proper and what is distant"*. Fischler (1988), when dealing with individual identity, emphasizes the mechanism of incorporation that is established in the relationship between the individual and food, which takes place in two spheres, concomitantly and synchronously: in the biological sphere, when the individual absorbs the food (nutrients) and in the cultural sphere, when he is absorbed by the food, in other words, incorporated with values, beliefs and representations of a historical and symbolic circulation.

Food tradition is not something innate in the individual; inculcation begins in childhood from the experiences gained from the tactile, gustatory and olfactory sensations of the food consumed (CANESQUI; GARCIA, 2005). However, in the contemporary era, several authors point out that this tradition is being shaken by commercial pressures and the pace of everyday life (HAWKES, 2002; CONTRERAS; GRACIA, 2011).

From a totalizing perspective, food is a biological and sociocultural manifestation. The biological element is limited to nutrition, i.e. the nutritional requirements for the optimal functioning of the human organism; while the sociocultural element is evident in food choices, which are not exclusively subject to economic motivations, although they are strongly determined by them (CONTRERAS; GRACIA, 2011), but also by their capacity to represent social meanings (CANESQUI; GARCIA, 2005). This is what makes it possible for different eating behaviors to coexist in different societies.

It is worth noting that the consolidation of these behaviors takes place in circumstances of tension, conflict and pacts, and has the following repercussions: they mark ethnic and social similarities and differences, classify and rank people and groups, express conceptions of the world and incorporate a great power of symbolic evocation (CONTRERAS; GRACIA, 2011).

Food plays an important role as a social marker that is easily identifiable. This is revealed by the type, quantity, aesthetics, way food items are arranged and the way they are consumed. These aspects constitute the distinguishing features between individuals and groups. When food styles are reshaped, this can mean a strategy to reach higher levels on the social ladder or even social ascension itself, as a way of becoming identical to the "others" in the group.

Even at the dawn of the 21st century, under the accelerated pace of globalization, the dichotomy in the field of food consumption by populations remains fierce (FAO, 2013), revealing a polarization between those who live with abundance and diversity of food, and others who lack food - in quantitative and qualitative terms - to meet their primary needs. However, malnutrition can be found in these two poles, expressing opposing morbid effects due to malnutrition or food shortages.

Over the years, problems relating to quality have been added to the traditional lack of equitable distribution of food, due to the different types of health risks associated with it, such as food-borne illnesses and obesity and other related chronic diseases. According to Contreras (2005), this has led to a redefinition of the concept of food safety to counter the dietary dictates that govern the dominant social logic. It is now based on three pillars:

access to food as a human right, food guarantees in qualitative and quantitative terms and food practices that are consistent with cultural traditions and environmentally sustainable (MALUF, 2007).

With this concept in mind, it is worth highlighting some of the social facts that are threatening intangible heritage, which is made up of beliefs, cuisine and consumption habits, constituted by food multiculturalism. As a result, cultural food traditions can become destabilized and even extinct over time.

In recent years, several articles have reported on trends in industrialized countries towards the homogenization of food consumption (CONTRERAS; GRACIA, 2011; GARCIA, 2003), drastic changes in consumption patterns and eating habits in the developing world (UUSITALLO; PIETINEN; PEKKA, 2002) and an increase in the worldwide incidence of diet-related diseases (CHOPRA, 2002; WHO, 2003b), bringing to light a new problem in the field of food. This arises in a scenario where there is accelerated urbanization, technological modernization, greater participation of women in the labour market, concomitant with the increased concentration and power of large corporations that cheapen their products and integrate them into the international market. All this is having an impact on the global health of this and future generations (UUSITALLO; PIETINEN; PEKKA, 2002).

As we have seen, it is at the heart of these socio-political and economic changes that food multiculturalism is losing its solidity. Bourdieu (2001) states that cultural goods in contemporary neoliberal society are endangered by the driving force of the market and food culture fits perfectly into his analysis. The author points out that, firstly, we must dispel the illusion that technological innovations and economic ventures increase the quantity and quality of cultural goods on offer and consumer satisfaction, as advocated by the defenders of capital, because what is actually circulating is a commodity for profit and indifferent to ties with history or the identity of a group. Secondly, it is also necessary to break with the myth that the extraordinary differentiation and diversification of products is opposed to the standardization of supply, both on a national and international scale, because competition does not diversify - but homogenizes - in search of products that are acceptable to the "maximum public" in all countries. In conclusion, the author argues that it is necessary to reinforce that the logic of profit, especially short-term profit, is the strict negation of culture.

Faced with the prospect of cultural homogenization triggered by globalization, imposing obstacles against the dissolution of food multiculturalism, understood as the intertwining of symbolic and cultural practices introjected by individuals in the sphere of food, can have a positive impact both in the gastronomic field and in terms of health benefits. This is because the existence of a variety of food preparations made up of healthy foods makes it possible to achieve a nutritional balance in the diet and promote health.

Undoubtedly, it is the transnational expansion of food corporations with their multiple sustainability strategies that leads to the destruction of the food base, the loss of biodiversity and food insecurity, thus contributing to the destruction of local food culture (PHILLIPS, 2006). The links between industry and the countryside, under the dominance of the former, linking the guarantee of the purchase of the product to strict compliance with technical production requirements, has dismantled small-scale agricultural production, causing it to lose its diversity and autonomy in growing traditional foods. This is because the oligopoly that governs the global food system, according to Stuckler & Nestle (2012), dictates what you eat and how you eat it.

In this way, the advent of the obesity pandemic is one of the signs of the contradictions of this global business model. The obvious association between energy-dense diets and obesity and other comorbidities makes it possible to identify Westernized diet styles as risk factors for this disease (CHOPRA, 2002; WHO, 2003b). From there, concern arose about carbonated drinks and fast foods, which are the driving forces of American global corporations. Such products are becoming more prevalent in the global diet, largely due to the intensive penetration of multinationals in countries, including within the emerging markets of large urban centers in middle- and low-income countries (HAWKES, 2002).

As a result of urbanization, Gracia (2005) states that the daily diet of the contemporary diner has undergone substantial changes: meals are now structured by time, socialized only in leisure conditions, replaced by *snacks* in situations of intense work activity and, when eaten at home, are made up of industrialized products. Forced to rationalize time and deal with the stressful circumstances of work (distances, schedules, transport), eating out in restaurants, cafés and bars, including *fast food*, is the norm for many individuals.

Ultra-processed products stand out in the world of unhealthy industrialized foodstuffs. They are products derived from industrialized ingredients, made up of oils, fats, starches and sugars, as well as an association of additives to make them palatable (MONTEIRO, 2009; MONTEIRO et al, 2013). This creates a mixture that mimics the taste and smell of the food, allowing consumers to recognize it as an edible product. Products of this nature, with an unbalanced nutritional composition, high in calories and low in strategic nutrients and highly stimulating to consume, are the ones that have negative effects on health. In the view of Monteiro & Cannon (2012), these products are just as harmful to health as cigarettes and alcohol, despite their particularities.

With the emergence of *fast-food*, fast-consumption foods are offered in practical packaging and, in general, are nutritionally unbalanced, but in keeping with the restricted pace and time imposed on meals. It is the type of food preferred by teenagers, distributed by large commercial chains, including transnational ones, which use aggressive marketing strategies - associating its consumption with an image of elevated social *status* and a modern lifestyle - to create demands and consolidate changes in eating habits (HAWKES, 2002).

Garcia (2003) calls this context "contemporary commensality", especially due to the scarcity of time to prepare and consume food and the abundant and diversified supply of food items that can be prepared quickly. This is what is shaping the eating habits of industrialized countries (CONTRERAS, 2005) and emerging countries (HAWKES, 2002), in a very accelerated way, thanks to the reinforced advertising and marketing strategies of food companies that overshadow cultural references.

For consumers to establish bonds of belonging with industrialized food, they need to fill the "void" inherent in the artificialized product and bring it closer to the edible elements of nature. However, technology is increasingly making this product less identifiable to the sense organs, due to its modified organoleptic characteristics, the wrapping that contains it, and it is reduced to its appearance and representation, despite the industries' efforts to mask it so that it resembles natural food. For FISCHLER (1998), the modern consumer's lack of knowledge about how food is produced, its origin and history creates a situation of discomfort dominated by uncertainty, mistrust and anxiety.

However, the criticism of industrialized food products goes beyond their impact on traditional food practices and representations. It is known that the introduction of food products into people's eating routines is not the result of strictly rational choices, but is influenced by the dynamic social context of everyday life, which conditions these choices (DELORMIER; FROHLICH; POTVIN, 2009). The crux of the problem is that there is a special set of food products, widely offered and widely consumed by the world's population, completely artificialized, intensely advertised, involved in a series of health hazards, of very low cost, unbalanced nutritional composition, with commercial transit devoid of regulatory barriers and high profitability for transnational companies. These products pose a high risk to global health, given their involvement in the obesity pandemic and associated CNCDs (WHO, 2002a). These are the so-called unhealthy food products (WHO, 2003b), a designation that will be used throughout this work and whose attributes will be explored in later chapters.

Food can have multiple effects on the lives of individuals and communities, bringing them closer to or further away from cultural traits, health profiles and psychosocial balance. The globalization of the food market releases barriers to allow the free transit of its products and disrespects the diversity of the food culture of population groups. It is also able to eliminate any obstacle that contradicts its purpose of "mass consumption," rationalization of the production process and concealment of social differences. In short, it acts by removing any obstacle to the logic of this economic model in order to increase its profits.

Thus, the way forward is to revitalize local food styles, including in strategic consumption spaces (community restaurants, school canteens, nurseries, among others), as a way of rescuing the symbolic value of food and reducing the possibility of dispersal of histories and cultures, as well as the risk of disease, as a result of predatory market practices. Any incentive for changes that allow a return to a balanced diet, mixed with natural, healthy and culturally acceptable foods, carried out in a sharing environment, is valid for regaining this cultural-food value, associated with health and, therefore, improved quality of life.

2.2 The diverse panorama of food risks

The social dynamics that drive transformations in the food production and marketing system have numerous repercussions, despite increasing food availability (WHO, 2000). Among these repercussions are the maintenance of high poverty rates in certain regions of the planet (FAO, 2013a), changes to people's lifestyles and daily eating practices, and the intensification and diversification of food risks (WHO, 2003b). These facts have destabilized individual and collective health conditions over the decades. The adverse effects stem from the characteristics of the food and/or the intensity of its consumption, measured in terms of quantity, quality and the combination of both. Based on these parameters, it is possible to synthetically characterize three major groups of risks that affect the health of the community: hunger/ malnutrition, food-borne diseases and obesity/ chronic non-communicable diseases - CNCDs.

With regard to the risk of hunger/ malnutrition, it can be seen that it is a social phenomenon that has accompanied the history of humanity, practically confined to groups socially excluded by the economic model and living in different regions of the world. This problem does not lie in the inability of world food production to supply the planet's population (FAO, 2011a), but in the global food production and distribution system itself, which is not committed to meeting everyone's basic nutritional needs.

According to FAO estimates, around 925 million people on the planet are food insecure, concentrated in sub-Saharan Africa, Asia and the Pacific, regions deeply affected by the economic crisis and the food crisis of 2007/2008 (FAO, 2010). The shortage of food resulting from this crisis meant that stocks were insufficient to meet the food demand of the entire population, which was reflected in the fact that the number of undernourished people in Asia remained practically stable. However, in Africa, the number of undernourished people increased, given its dependence on imports, the unavailability of sufficient food stocks and budgetary resources to adequately protect the food security of the most vulnerable (FAO, 2011b).

As for child malnutrition, the recent global panorama drawn up by the *Save the Children Fund* (2012) reveals that 90% of the world's malnourished children are concentrated in 36 countries; it is estimated that 170 million of them suffer from chronic malnutrition and more than 2.6 million die each year from this disease. The persistence of hunger and malnutrition results from inadequate access to food due to lack of income, the poor condition of socially excluded and economically marginalized individuals (FAO, 2012), and is a reflection of the structural conditions of society. Despite this bleak scenario, over the decades from the 1960s to the 1990s, there was a 10% drop in the total number of people in developing countries who had a daily diet of less than 2100 calories *per capita* (SEIPEL, 1999), although several hundred million people in the world still have their survival threatened.

In Brazil, the comparative results of national surveys[10] carried out between the 1970s and 1990s showed that there was a 72% decline in the prevalence of child malnutrition (BATISTA FILHO & RISSIN, 2003). Meanwhile, food and nutritional security social policies, implemented at the beginning of this millennium, were fundamental in reducing poverty and simultaneously improving nutritional status, since over 20 million people

10 In Brazil, three nationwide surveys were carried out during this period: the National Study of Family Expenditure (ENDEF) in 1974/75; the National Health and Nutrition Survey (PNSN) in 1989; and the National Demographic and Health Survey (PNDS) in 1995/96.

were lifted out of poverty between 2003 and 2009 (DEL GROSSI, 2010). These effects are reflected in the low prevalence of chronic malnutrition (height deficit) in children under 5 years of age, whose values reached 6.3% and 5.7%, respectively, for males and females (BRASIL; IBGE, 2010). As a result, this disease is no longer considered a public health problem in Brazil, according to the WHO classification[11] (WHO, 2013a).

The **first group of risks** in the contemporary era include food-borne diseases - FBDs[12], which are analyzed only in relation to food products and meals outside the home, which correspond to the new eating practices adopted in a context of urbanization. It is therefore a question of mapping the different risks posed by food vehicles, at local and international level, and the impacts on health.

In 1984, the WHO considered ATDs to be one of the most widespread public health problems in the contemporary world. These diseases are responsible for causing social and economic impacts, due to the consequences in terms of illness, death and/or disability; the condemnation, rejection and loss of products, affecting the international market; and the reduction in tourism activities (WHO, 1984). Food safety concerns consist of avoiding biological contamination (microorganisms, parasites), physical contamination and chemical contamination (residues of additives, pesticides, biotoxins), by controlling the critical points of the entire production chain, which can be done through technical qualification, the application of control methods, regular sanitary inspections, food education, among other measures.

Almost 40 years on, climate change appears not only to have the potential to reduce food supplies, but also to increase the toxic and microbial contamination of food (HALL, D'SOUZA & KIRK, 2002). At the same time, the improvement of food production and manufacturing technologies is accelerating, aimed at creating and diversifying inputs and products, increasing agricultural profitability, expanding the product distribution network, as well as other economic benefits, with a view to increasing productivity, expanding business and the capital gains of companies and their conglomerates.

In this context, different causal agents have emerged, including unusual modalities,

11 The WHO considers malnutrition to be a public health problem when it affects 20% or more of the population.

12 ATDs include diarrheal diseases caused by food contamination due to unsanitary living conditions (housing without drinking water, sewage disposal, cold equipment, etc.) combined with limited information on hygiene. In English, these illnesses are referred to as *Foodborne* diseases, defined as illnesses caused by eating food contaminated by pathogenic microorganisms, chemical contaminants and biotoxins (WHO, 2007).

causing diseases with severe and rare symptoms, as was the case with the prions responsible for Bovine Spongiform Encephalopathy (BSE), a fatal neurodegenerative disease diagnosed in 1996 in the United Kingdom (WHO, 1999), where 39 cases were recorded. Also in 1994, an already known bacterial agent became a new emerging pathogen, *E. Coli* O157:H7, which caused an outbreak in the United States (ARMSTRONG, HOLLINGSWORTH & GLENN MORRIS, 1996), and later there was another notable outbreak involving improperly cooked hamburger (KING et al, 2009).

According to Weiss & McMichael (2004), the multiplicity of effects of globalization, such as the process of accentuated urbanization, the growth of dense and precarious peripheral residential areas, an increase in the volume of trade, a change in consumer habits, the invasion of natural environments for agricultural exploitation, climate change and massive technological development, create a scenario that encourages new contacts between wildlife and humans and facilitates cross-infection between species, triggering the risk of spreading emerging infectious diseases.

The intense pace of international food trade does not always result in benefits for the community, as it increases the risk of infectious diseases being transmitted across borders, since food simultaneously has two important characteristics: being the main commercial *commodity* and an excellent vehicle for transmitting diseases (KAFERSTEIN, MOTARJEMI & BETTCHER, 1997). Thus, transcontinental outbreaks involving semi-processed and processed products are frequently recorded (TAUXE, 1996; HALL, D'SOUZA & KIRK, 2002). Products such as imported peanuts contaminated with salmonella spread outbreaks in four countries on three different continents, triggering an international alert (KIRK et al, 2004). An outbreak of hepatitis A due to contaminated frozen strawberries was the result of production shared between two countries (HUTIN et al, 1999). New foods are now beginning to be implicated in outbreaks, such as seed sprouts, which are incorporated into eating habits (TAORMINA, BEUCHAT & SLUTSKER, 1999).

In this context, food has already proved that it can be a potential source of risk, not only because it harbors microorganisms or pathogenic particles and carries chemical contaminants, such as pollutants and pesticides, but also because of the intrinsic changes generated by new technologies, which have given rise to genetically modified foods, or which cause antimicrobial resistance in biological agents (SCALLAN, 2007).

As for industrial development, certain economic activities generate persistent organic pollutants - POPs - which include many organochlorine pesticides, industrial chemicals and by-products of certain industrial processes, as well as incineration residues. These are polychlorinated biphenyls, dioxins and furans - substances that are highly harmful to health and can persist in the soil, sediments and deposits of these wastes for decades and even centuries, as well as being carried over long distances by global air and water currents. These sources of pollutants, both historical and current, contaminate the animal and human food chain, animal feed, eggs, chicken, fish and seafood, as has been documented in certain European countries (WHO, 2014). Food is therefore the main source of human exposure to these contaminants (WEBER et al, 2008).

A study on the diet of the American food basket, made up of fresh and processed foods, found that POP residues were present in 10% of the samples and that they also contained residues of dieldrin. In addition, residues of DDT (dichlorodiphenyltrichloroethane) and its metabolites were present in more than 20% of the samples tested in 1998 and 1999, both insecticides banned since the early 1970s (SCHAFER; KEGLEY, 2002). According to the WHO technical report (2003a), this group of substances can cause serious effects such as cancer, altered immune function, reproductive dysfunction, neurological alterations and physical development.

With regard to genetically modified foods, some studies have concluded that, although this technology applied to food expands production capacity, it presents potential risks that require further research to confirm their health safety (BAKSHI, 2003; COSTA et al, 2011). As for health effects, Bakshi (2003) highlights food allergies and other effects due to exposure to the new proteins introduced in these foods, and antimicrobial resistance due to the recombination of genes from this food with those of pathogenic bacteria, either in the environment or in the intestinal tract of the diner. These were some of the reasons that made up the arsenal of arguments for Europe's rejection of Novartis BT corn.

Bacterial resistance in food-borne pathogens is another international concern. As a result, the *Codex Alimentarius* (FAO; WHO, 2005) has approved a code of practice aimed at minimizing the adverse effects on public health resulting from the use of microbial agents in food produced from animals. In Morocco, the analysis of 11,516 samples distributed among beef, chicken, water and seafood, pepper, among others, revealed that 105 (0.91%) of them were positive for *Salmonella* and 25 of them showed resistance to at least one antimicrobial tested (BOUCHRIF et al, 2009).

Although eating fruit and vegetables is an option that is valued because it is a type of healthy consumption, these foods are not without risks. In Brazil, the analytical results of a total of 2,488 fruit and vegetable samples analyzed in 2010 revealed that 35% of them contained residues, due to non-compliance with the grace periods specified for the correct use of the pesticide; 28% contained residues of unauthorized pesticides or, if authorized, exceeded the maximum permitted limits. Furthermore, of the total of 18 foods sampled, five - peppers, cucumbers, strawberries, carrots and lettuce - showed condemnation equal to or greater than 50% of the total category analyzed (BRASIL; ANVISA, 2011). These results suggest that the population is exposed to various risks and persistent complications, considering the type of agent in question (WHO, 2002b).

This current scenario, permeated with food risks from extrinsic, traditional and unusual causal agents, producing diverse, acute and chronic morbid effects, seems likely to continue and increase over the years, as they reflect the antagonisms of the global economic model. In addition, in the last decades of the 20th century, there was the global obesity epidemic, which has a direct relationship with food and has now become a major threat to public health due to the comorbidities involved (WHO, 2000; VISSCHER; SEIDELL, 2001).

Obesity is a chronic disease with a largely preventive nature (WHO, 2004a), caused both by a sedentary lifestyle and by the consumption of unhealthy, energy-dense diets which, together, form a highly "obesogenic" environment, unbalancing the energy balance of individuals and contributing to excessive weight gain (PRENTICE, 2005, WHO, 2000; PINHEIROS, FREITAS; CORSO, 2004; CABALLERO, 2007).

This establishes the link between diet and the etiology of obesity, as well as other chronic non-communicable diseases (CHOPRA, 2002). In fact, it is special types of industrialized food, already defined above, which, by systematically participating in the habitual diet, contribute to health disorders (WHO, 2004a).

This creates the **second group of** current food **risks** - the focus of this paper - in which an important causal factor is intrinsically linked to the nutritional composition of food products. Risks that do not derive from the introduction of a biological, chemical or physical agent, which is carried from the outside into the food product, but which is intrinsic to its very formula and identity. Risks that challenge this new century because they raise tensions between the freedom of transnational economic agents to create profitable food products and the need to commit to preserving society's health.

These are products derived from a global food market, which has developed artifices to cater for a large audience in urban metropolises, with reduced production costs, through the use of less noble ingredients in the composition of foods, such as fats and sugars, making them foods with a high energy density and nutritionally poor (POPKIN; GORDON-LARSEN, 2004; MONTEIRO, 2009; UUSITALO; PIETIENEN; PUSKA, 2002). These unhealthy products are surrounded by an advertising apparatus that occupies the different spaces of everyday life to encourage individuals to take an interest in this type of food consumption (HARRIS et al, 2009).

In short, the food economy, driven by globalization, has varied and contradictory effects that have a direct impact on society. There are benefits, on the one hand, brought about by the increase in the availability of food and the expansion of its variety (WHO, 2002), and disadvantages, on the other, such as the marketing of unhealthy and unsafe products (ROBERTSON, 2001; FAO, 2013b). This set of characteristics increases and diversifies the risks to health, either through the growing loss of nutritional quality (WHO, 2004a, 2003b), or through compromised health quality (WHO, 2006), or even simultaneously through these two dimensions, with manifestations at local and global levels.

Thus, there is an urgent need for local and international measures towards a comprehensive and dynamic approach to food risks that are capable of incorporating health and nutritional aspects into quality management measures; promoting intersectoral coordination between bodies that have an interface with food and health; and mobilizing other interested parties - society and the market - with a view to changing the current epidemiological situation.

2.3 Health risks: from a mathematical concept to a socio-political and cultural construction

The notion of risk was commonly used in the 16th and 17th centuries to deal with the misadventures of nature during the maritime exploration expeditions undertaken by Western peoples (GIDDENS, 2010). Risks had to be predicted, even if they were based on restricted references and below the "sea" of the unknown, so that the advantages and disadvantages could be weighed up and decisions made about the feat. Since then, analyzing risks has involved uncertainties, calculations, analysis and positioning.

Now, "risk" has been used in different fields of knowledge to predict both natural and socially created events. With its application, the ideas of space and time have been added to those of uncertainty and have come to make up the notion of risk (GIDDENS, 2010). The analysis of a given "risk" phenomenon involves probabilistic calculations, based on the combination of a set of factors that simplify the complex reality in which it regularly occurs, while always remaining overshadowed by uncertainties.

In fact, risk is not an entity in itself; its existence depends on the characterization of the danger or unwanted event (EWALD, 1991). Risk and danger are therefore interrelated and, at the same time, differentiated. The former is an objective threat, while the latter is the event itself or the presence of the causal agent triggering the event. However, this distinction is completely annulled in the absence of alternatives or possibilities for risk-free action, in which case risk is danger (LUHMANN, 1993).

In contemporary society, the technical-industrial transformations fostered by the articulation between science and technology have driven the accelerated updating and reformulation of goods, products and services to meet the demand induced by the consumer market and, consequently, to expand capital (BAUMAN, 1999; BECK, 2002). A type of economic rationality prevails which focuses unilaterally on increasing productivity and profits and neglects the risks linked to this (BECK, 2002).

It is in this context of capitalist development that new forms of social risk emerge as a reflexive effect of the technological process, which intensify and diversify on an individual and collective level (GIDDENS, 1991; BECK, 2002). According to Giddens (1991), this technological reflexivity is due to the inability to control the complex set of factors involved in concrete reality, when applying scientific knowledge and technological innovations in practice. In these circumstances, risks are those factors that arise unexpectedly, or rather, deviations from the norm.

It is important to point out that these deviations that escape control cannot be reported as a limitation of scientific knowledge, as they are risks consistent with the intrinsic nature of knowledge itself (NARDOCCI, 2002). According to the author, the truth is that knowledge is always approximate when exploring a given object in a dynamic and complex social reality.

However, this instability of scientific discoveries, which always progress in situations of uncertainty, especially when it comes to risks, revealing the changing nature of science, is what gave rise to the Precautionary Principle. This instrument is based on the adoption of protective measures against risks, even if there is no reliable scientific data about them (GIDDENS, 2010). Thus, in the absence of a scientific explanation to support the decision and the consequences of the imputed risks, the political meanings they take on become explicit (CARAPINHEIRO, 2002), delineated by the advantages and benefits attributed to those who produced them.

In this sense, risk comes to be approached in an ambiguous way (BECK, 2002; GIDDENS, 2010), representing, on the one hand, the boldness, challenge and economic dynamism of society in its quest for productivity and progress and, on the other, the effects of technological impulses that materialize in the form of damage, harm and threats, in a social and material sense.

However, from the perspective of the dominant neoliberal doctrine, risks are a constituent element of life. The norm is generalized competition, and the expected behavior of companies and individuals is to overcome, which depends on the ability to remove obstacles within the possibilities, adopting certain precautions. This rules out any possibility of claiming the impartiality of science and technology (BODSTEIN, 2000), since both are duly supported by solid political-ideological foundations. In addition to this, it should be emphasized that risks presuppose, at the other extreme, benefits, understood as advantages or profits extracted from economic activity (NARDOCCI, 2002), despite the possible adverse effects on health or the environment arising from this activity.

For Luhmann (1993), "risk" and "danger" are attributes of the precarious regularity of life in society and emerge primarily from human activity. Their presence denotes possibilities of failure, failure or inability to eliminate causal agents, which can result in illness and death. This points to the conflicting nature of risk: sometimes it is something that needs constant control and sometimes it is something whose acceptance maintains the dynamism of the economy and society. As risks carry with them instability and uncertainty, imposing the need to make judgments and choices, i.e. political decisions (NARDOCCI, 2002), they become a socio-cultural construction (CARAPINHEIRO, 2002).

These premises influenced the development of the concepts of risk and hazard established by the FAO & WHO (FAO; WHO, 2005) and which are applied in the context of food health control. Thus, risk is the probability of an adverse health effect occurring as a result of the presence of one or more hazards in food; hazard is the presence of the causal agent in the food, responsible for this effect. From these concepts, two considerations can be drawn: firstly, this conception treats the phenomenon in a reductionist way, in which the "social" is removed from the scene so that the biological sciences seek the support of mathematical knowledge, placing this knowledge as central to the construction of the concept; and secondly, the complex and dynamic reality, rationalized in numbers, creates an image that it is possible to control the unpredictable whole. Carapinheiro (2002) informs us that it is this supposed neutrality of the term "risk", based on probabilistic calculations, and without mentioning the social character present in its formation, that makes it preferable to the term "danger".

Thus, when the technical-scientific apparatus is applied to food and turns it into a potential object of risk, two effects can arise in the sphere of food health control: the current one, recognized from both international and national perspectives, which is the risk of food attributed predominantly to biological, chemical or physical agents in food (FAO; WHO, 2005), due to epidemic outbreaks and intoxications, and the negative impacts on health and trade (KATZ et al, 1999; KAFERSTEIN et al, 1997), due to contaminated food (WHO, 2006). And the emerging one, which is linked to the intrinsic nature of the formula of the food product, which results in the excessive presence of certain components (sugars, fats, additives and salt), when an unbalanced nutritional quality is evident, being associated with the obesity pandemic and other CNCDs (MONTEIRO, 2010; WHO, 2004a; DREWNOWSKI, 2009; POPKIN, 2001).

In this way, the growing and different risks arising from technological innovations - and the complexity of identifying them - constitute the challenge of modernity, not only because of the economic and social damage caused to society, but also because of the distrust in the quality of food and the insecurity generated in the consumption of products. In addition, Hespanha (2002) states that these far-reaching risks place the onus of responsibility on public authorities to circumvent the deviations generated by "industrial progress". He also reports that the factors of uncertainty and unpredictability that are created and recreated around them increase the obstacles to effective intervention by surveillance and control systems.

In view of this, and as a consequence of the risks, there has been a strong push to create new surveillance and control systems and to expand the regulatory action of public authorities (BODSTEIN, 2000). These systems require a body of specialized experts with the technical competence to make decisions on how to intervene in risks and restore safety. Credibility and trust depend exclusively on the performance of these systems (GIDDENS, 1991).

As the discussion of risks and intervention measures affects collective well-being, citizens are urged to participate in the decision-making process to establish the degree of market freedom and social acceptability of risks (NARDOCCI, 2002). In view of this, the FAO & WHO (2005) recommend that government bodies enter into partnerships with the different social forces involved - the market, consumers and universities - in order to trigger the risk analysis process.

For this reason, in order to establish safety limits, the biological component and the social component always come together in the process of analyzing food risks. The former is defined from the technical-scientific apparatus that justifies the characteristics and potential of the danger involved, through pathogenicity, virulence, mutagenicity, toxicity, among other types of expression of harmfulness (FAO, 1995). As for the second, the scientific knowledge that underpins the interpretation of risks, combined with the context of socio-political implications, determines whether or not they are accepted. Depending on the underlying social processes, risks can be reduced or intensified, becoming a social issue (BECK, 2002), since it is a phenomenon of multiple contingency that offers different observers a range of perspectives on the impacts in terms of loss or damage (LUHMANN, 1993).

In view of the above, this involvement of heterogeneous social forces in dealing with the issue shows that the findings on risk result from the combination of the technical-scientific component and socio-political interests, which determine the impacts on social, political and economic costs and benefits. In this context, Beck (2002) argues that science takes on the social and political significance of risk, through decisions on the content of knowledge and effects, the scope and type of danger, the public affected in the long term, liability, rights to claim compensation, etc.

Today, the concept of "food safety" is under question because, with its restricted scope and inability to cover all the recognized risks of food, it is not possible to guarantee that food promotes and maintains health. It is therefore essential to include emerging risks, those that contribute to overweight disorders and their comorbidities, in the concept and practice that govern control systems, so that they are compatible with the reality of the nutritional profile. This mismatch between the adjustments made by the control institutions and the speed at which risks emerge is due to both technical difficulties and political obstacles. And this slow and limited capacity of institutional action to encompass the diversity of food risks has a direct impact on the health of the exposed population. Thus, the expansion of the field of "monitoring food risks", including health and nutritional aspects, is mainly dependent on the support of specialists who, through their technical, scientific and political foundations, will stimulate a change in institutional conduct.

In view of this, and based on Beck's (2002) argument, foods with attributes such as "healthy" and "safe" are difficult and complex to prove in the current social order. For the author, the food risks that challenge humanity can only be identified through sophisticated resources and limited access, as they are no longer expressed in the way they once were. As the sense organs are insufficient to capture them, individual autonomy to defend oneself is compromised. According to this author, the systemic damage caused by risks encompasses all living beings, and humans are affected without distinction of class, ethnicity or gender, being completely unprotected by the permeability of national state borders, which no longer impose obstacles in an interconnected social environment.

Although the risks relate to the collective, the effects are socially stratified. Individuals differ in their degree of exposure. Those who are socially vulnerable,

because they are deprived of symbolic and material resources for their defense and self-protection, are the most intensely affected by the consequences of risks. This can be seen in the relationship between the consumption of high-risk foods and obesity in a poverty-stricken environment (MARTINS, 2007; DREWNOWSKI & SPECTER, 2004; WHO, 2000).

In short, the risks and dangers generated by accelerated industrialization do not derive from the responsibility of conscious personal choices, as is attributed to the consumption of cigarettes, food products or alcoholic beverages, the control of which depends on individual behaviour or self-control. These risks are structurally constructed (PETERSON & LUPTON, 2000). As the configuration of risks is complex, allowing for only limited scientific evidence and imprecise effects, the position on their acceptance is a key element of the analysis process and, regardless of whether the risk is characterized as individual or collective, it is mediated by a set of political-ideological and cultural interests on what is recognized as a risk. In general, conflicting interests form the basis of reference for weightings, the result of which will reflect the flexibility or rigidity of the commitment made to the health of the collective.

The effective defence of society is primarily in the hands of citizens, preferably in an organized way, and it is up to them to monitor food risks and those who control these risks - the official institutions. However, for this to happen, citizens need to make an effort to get hold of information and win the spaces that will allow them to voice their needs and intervene in the decisions of the competent bodies. However, they must always be careful not to shy away from highlighting the submerged structural issues of society, which decisively shape production-consumption patterns and gradually deteriorate the health of the community.

3 FOOD PRODUCTS AND HEALTH: A MULTIFACETED ANALYSIS

3.1 Food products and health risks: the view of intergovernmental organizations

3.1.1 The WHO and FAO approach to the issue

Successive documents have been published by the WHO since the end of the 1980s, announcing to the world the global impacts of new food consumption practices and sedentary lifestyles on the health of the public, especially those in urbanized regions. In 1989, in its document "*Diet, Nutrition and Prevention of Chronic Disease*", the WHO mobilized to warn that the consumption of unhealthy food products has become one of the factors responsible for triggering a range of chronic diseases, which are spreading in ascending proportions in the population, such as obesity, cardiovascular diseases and various types of cancer. Considering the multifactorial causality of these diseases and the crucial importance of the way we eat, the WHO advocates that this food-disease binomial should be the subject of intersectoral public health and nutrition policies (WHO, 1990).

This WHO document is the initial milestone in the analysis of the global repercussions of changes in dietary patterns, technological innovations in the field of food production and lifestyles, among other aspects, on the epidemiological profile of countries on several continents. On that occasion, he pointed out that the dynamics resulting from the economic development model are leading these nations to "reproduce" some of the cultural and social characteristics of the rich countries, especially those of the United States of America, as the greatest exponent of the industrial-consumerist project, such as the frenetic consumption pattern, the automation of customary activities and the morbidity profile.

In the year 2000, the WHO focused on exploring the most obvious effect of this change in diet and lifestyle on health and published a specific technical report on obesity, entitled "*Obesity: preventing and managing the global epidemic*". It recognized obesity as a chronic epidemic disease, of a global and preventive nature, caused by dietary factors and patterns of physical activity, highlighting food products circulating worldwide as one of the causal agents. With this, it recommended to governments, among other intervention measures, the need to reformulate food regulations with regard to quality requirements, safety, labeling and food advertising (WHO, 2004a).

This highlighted the fundamental role of governments, without excluding the responsibility of industries, in intervening in the food market. This is because this market is completely undisciplined in terms of meeting nutritional quality requirements. The use of formulations with an excess of caloric and non-nutritive ingredients, which contribute to the appearance of diseases in the individuals who consume these products, are examples of factors that should be regulated.

The exclusively positive image of food products that the media has consistently conveyed, as symbols of innovation and creativity, versatility in meeting consumer needs, the strength of the industry and the global market, practicality of consumption, among others, is beginning to be deconstructed. These factors are also increasingly being identified for their dissonant effects with the precepts of health promotion and maintenance. In short, they are revealed as agents that contribute to long-term, highly complex illnesses. This situation calls for urgent curbs and regulations by health institutions.

Two years later, the WHO released the document "*Reducing Risks, Promoting Healthy Life*", in which it continued to emphasize the relationship between the consumption of unhealthy foods, such as *fast food* or processed and hypercaloric foods, and changes in lifestyle, with the diversified picture of diseases. It adds a new element to the discourse when it identifies the contradictions inherent in the process of economic globalization:

Globalization has been hailed as a strategy to reduce poverty, but the liberalization of trade can lead to both benefits and harms for health (p.6, Chapter One). The rapidly growing epidemic of noncommunicable diseases, already responsible for some 60% of world deaths, is clearly related to changes in global dietary patterns and increased consumption of industrially processed fatty, salty and sugary foods. Countries should give top priority to developing effective, committed policies for the prevention of globally increasing high risks to health, such as [...] unhealthy diet and obesity (p.11). They may [...] have to focus on [...] legislation to reduce the proportion of salt and other unhealthy components in foods; [...] (WHO, 2002a, *p.166*) .[13]

In addition, it points to the expansion of food trade - and its release policies - as stimulating the adoption of a diet based on the consumption of unhealthy processed foods by thousands of people. To this end, it recommends that governments prioritize the

13 Globalization is heralded as a strategy to reduce poverty, but trade liberalization can lead to both health benefits and harms (Chapter One, p.6). The growing epidemic of non-communicable diseases, already responsible for around 60% of the world's deaths, is clearly related to changes in global dietary patterns and the increased consumption of industrially processed foods rich in fatty acids, salt and sugar. Countries should prioritize the development of effective committed policies for the prevention of high global health risks, such as [...] unhealthy diet and obesity (p.11). They can [...] focus on [...] legislation to reduce the proportion of salt and other unhealthy components in foods; [...] (WHO, 2002a., p.166). (personal translation)

prevention of health risks (such as unhealthy diets), invest in legislation to reduce unhealthy food components and strengthen health promotion campaigns (WHO, 2002a).

Economic globalization has made it possible for food corporations to branch out around the world, distributing their products, changing people's culture in terms of eating habits and consumption practices and altering their nutritional and health profile. As can be seen from the above quote, food has changed to such an extent that it is possible to draw a line between "unhealthy" and "healthy" diets, depending on the foods that make up the diet, and the choice of one way or another to eat can be decisive in the path to health or illness.

In 2003, the FAO, considering its mission to deal with issues related to food and agricultural systems and the establishment of guidelines for food safety and nutritional adequacy, took a clearer stance on the binomial of NCDs and diets. It therefore combined its efforts with those of the WHO and published an updated version of the document *The Joint WHO/FAO Expert Consultation on diet, nutrition and the prevention of chronic diseases* (WHO, 2003b). The greatest value of this document consisted of explaining the evidence on the relationship between foods/nutrients and chronic diseases, as well as highlighting the impact of changes in the world food economy on dietary patterns, which showed an increase in the content of calories and saturated fats and a reduction in the amount of complex carbohydrates. As a result, these organizations reiterated the need to establish a dialogue with industries in order to adapt the formulation of food products to technically healthy parameters, as well as to intervene in the advertising of such products (FAO/WHO, 2003b).

According to this document, strategies in the field of food must look at the aspects of food safety and safe food together. The food must be adequate in terms of quantity and nutritional and health quality, i.e. proportional to the needs required by the individual or group, and at the same time it must meet a compatible health profile, which means the absence or presence of contaminants within the maximum permitted limits.

The advocacy in favor of reformulating the composition of industrialized products and limiting advertising about them will continue in WHO documents released in subsequent years. Considering that these food products are circulated globally, there is a clear limitation for countries to act alone in promoting healthy diets, which requires supranational coordination and governance. In this sense, this document points out the essential need to interfere in existing international standards that guide international trade, and explains the responsibility of the *Codex Alimentarius* Commission - CAC. [...] *The*

Codex Alimentarius - the intergovernmental standardsetting body through which nations agree on standards for food - is currently being reviewed. Its work in the area of nutrition and labelling could be further strengthened to cover diet- related aspects of health (WHO, 2003b, p.142)[14] . Despite being under the international leadership of the WHO and FAO, the *Codex* Commission, a strategic institution for dealing with the issue, was only mentioned a decade after these debates began.

As the epidemiological situation worsened, the WHO's institutional rhetoric improved in two ways: on the one hand, by decoding the types of target products and intervention measures more precisely and, on the other, by emphasizing the asymmetries of the trade liberalization policy and calling on governments to take action. The attribute of unhealthy was used in the documents to describe the category of hypercaloric food products (high in fats and/or simple sugars) and those with a high salt content. This treatment of this group of food products leads to a reduction in their symbolic value on the market and, on the other hand, encourages individuals to be cautious in their consumption and governments to interfere in the industry to improve food standards. However, the *Codex Alimentarius* itself seems to be shielding itself from dealing with the issue of the "nutritional quality of food", since so far there has been no explicit manifestation of initiatives to create a space for internal debate, and even less to revisit the standards and technical procedures it has issued, with a view to adjusting food products to a profile considered to be healthy.

In 2004, at its annual assembly, the WHO approved the *Global Strategy on Diet, Physical Activity and Health*, which reiterates the two main risk factors for chronic diseases, unhealthy diets and reduced physical activity, and defines measures to promote health and prevent and reduce these diseases, which contribute substantially to the global burden of morbidity, mortality and disability. To this end, it reaffirms the commitment and mobilization of different social actors - civil society, industry and government - with the latter playing a crucial role. In the field of food, it points out that government action should be directed towards: interfering in the formulation of food products, making them compatible with the precepts of a healthy diet; regulating the *marketing of* children's food; creating tax incentives for healthy consumption, among others. However, the highlight of this document is the intense reinforcement for the CAC to make efforts to minimize the

---

14 [...] The *Codex Alimentarius* - the intergovernmental standards body through which nations agree on food standards - is being reviewed. Its work in the area of nutrition and labeling could be strengthened to cover diet-related aspects of health (WHO, 2003b, p.142).

impact of marketing products with unhealthy dietary standards and to strengthen the development of production and processing standards that take into account the nutritional quality and safety of products. It also calls for the support of governments and organized civil society in this endeavor (WHO, 2004b).

[a]Prior to the World Health Assembly, the FAO, at its 18th Session of the Committee on Agriculture, examined, through its members, the documents *The Joint WHO/FAO Expert Consultation on Diet, nutrition and the prevention of chronic diseases* (FAO, 2004) and the draft WHO document *Global Strategy on Diet, Physical Activity and Health*. Despite the majority support for the recommendations contained in the WHO document (WHO, 2003b), they highlighted some aspects: the fragility of the scientific basis for establishing a causal relationship between food and NCDs; the importance of being flexible in the application of the global recommendations, taking into account the specific circumstances of each country; and the need to value food education to enable individuals and families to make conscious food choices (FAO, 2004).

As for the insufficient scientific basis of the study, this refers to the multiplicity of causal factors involved in diseases and the difficulty of pinpointing the isolated importance of a specific causal factor (food). However, the essential point has been made and is centered on the harmful effects on health resulting from the nutritional composition of unhealthy industrialized foods, which is the responsibility of the market and the object of government demands for control. With regard to the importance of "food education", although the subject is undoubtedly relevant, its role must always be put into perspective. As the proposal emerged in isolation from others that support a change in the logic of the food production and industrialization system, it seems to have the intention of simplifying the complexity of the health-disease process in question, trying to artificially reduce the solution to the problem to educating the population. Furthermore, "food education" alone is incapable of countering the powerful market mechanisms built up in an environment of extreme organization, if there are no other intervention strategies to discipline the market.

In 2012, recognizing the global threat of NCDs and the economic and social impacts that these diseases have on countries, the United Nations published the document "*Political Declaration of The High-Level Meeting of the General Assembly on the Prevention and Control of Non-communicable Diseases*" (UN, 2012), which highlights unhealthy diet, physical inactivity and obesity as risk factors that have a strong link with the four main

NCDs - cardiovascular diseases, cancer, chronic respiratory diseases and diabetes - and which are associated with the highest health costs and reduced productivity. The document therefore proposes that governments move forward with multisectoral interventions to reduce the risk factors for these diseases, through international agreements and strategies, education, legislation, regulatory and fiscal measures, involving all sectors of society. It explicitly mentions the need to promote interventions to reduce salt, sugar and saturated fats and eliminate *trans* fats in industrialized foods, as well as to discourage the production and marketing of foods that contribute to an unhealthy diet.

As a result, the WHO has proposed a Global Framework for Monitoring NCDs which includes 25 indicators and nine voluntary targets for their prevention and control, with a validity period of 2013-2020. Among the voluntary global targets that relate to the subject of this study is the goal of a 30% relative reduction in the population's average salt/sodium intake by 2025. In the group of indicators proposed for national systems, one of them aims to reduce the impact on children of the marketing of foods high in saturated fats, *trans* fats, free sugars or salt and non-alcoholic drinks. Another indicator proposes limiting saturated fat in the food supply (WHO, 2013b). As for sugar, nothing was mentioned.

More recently, the FAO has also shown itself to be very sensitive to the problems of excess weight, and has proposed a list of alternatives to encourage a healthy diet. It stated that, despite the fact that the modern production system makes it possible to expand the variety of products, this system strives to sell more ultra-processed foods, which contribute to excess weight. To this end, it has presented for discussion the strategies of taxing less nutritious products, nutrition education in schools and regulating food advertising to children (FAO, 2013b). Compared to the discussion in 2003, substantial progress was made in the field of valuing healthy eating and the commitment to intervene in overweight.

In short, over the last two decades, the understanding has become established that unhealthy industrialized products pose a high risk to health and should therefore be the object of intervention and control measures. However, the adoption of concrete measures aimed at reformulating the nutritional parameters of these products is still a long way off. This involves incorporating natural or semi-processed ingredients, but also complementary measures such as: highlighting warnings on labels to make consumers aware of the risks of consuming this type of product; differentiated price taxation to curb consumption of these products, etc. These are a series of measures which, for many national governments and intergovernmental bodies, still remain in the realm of intentions.

In a context of economic globalization, the links of dependence between nation-states and the intergovernmental bodies that regulate the international market are close and the action of these interlocutors, the WHO, FAO and the *Codex Alimentarius* Commission, is fundamental for dealing with this new risk of food products. Isolated action by national governments could trigger market retaliation and internal instability, since reformulating the nutritional profile of products implies costs for companies and a threat to their profits.

3.1.2 Codex Alimentarius' apathy towards new food risks

According to the documents presented above, the WHO and FAO issued several warnings and indications of the effects on the health of the global population caused by food products widely circulated on the international market. However, it took sixteen years, from 1990 to 2006, for the *Codex Alimentarius* Commission - CAC - to react, considering its responsibility to issue a code of reference standards for the national food control agencies of the member countries, industries, consumers and international trade (FAO; WHO, 2006a).

The implementation of the FAO/WHO Joint Food Standards Program is the responsibility of the CAC, which has among its purposes: *[...] (a) protecting the health of consumers and ensuring fair practices in the food trade; [...] (e) amending published standards, after appropriate survey in the light of developments*[15] (FAO; WHO, 2006b, p.14). The mission of protecting health against food risks already presupposes openness to an unknown event and, therefore, a willingness to adjust standards in the light of renewed scientific knowledge, according to the dynamism of society and the new risk situations that arise, in order to safeguard the health of consumers.

However, it can be seen that the focus of the CAC's regulations is limited to the health safety of food, which involves sanitary parameters, the establishment of contaminant limits and provisions on labeling, its central objective being to protect the health of consumers against the risks of DTA (FAO; WHO, 2006b). This restricts the space for other threats that fall outside its scope - the nutritional components of unhealthy food products

15 [...] (a) protect the health of consumers and ensure fair practices in the food trade; [...] (e) adjust to published standards, after appropriate examination in the light of development (FAO;WHO, 2006a, p.14). [Personal translation]

- even though they are part of the universe of food risks that compromise society worldwide.

Thus, it was only in 2006 that the CAC launched an action plan to implement the *Global Strategy on Diet, Physical Activity and Health*, in which it recognized the affinity between its own mission and the strategies of this document, since nutrients associated with a high risk of NCDs had been identified (FAO; WHO, 2006a). This was based on the *Codex* mandate, which provides for measures to minimize the consumption of these nutrients in order to prevent consumer health disorders, as well as to guarantee the use of nutritional *claims* that are not false or confusing. As a result, the task was delegated to two specific *Codex* Committees, one dealing with matters relating to nutrition and foods for special dietary purposes (FAO; WHO, 2013), and the other dealing with food labeling (FAO; WHO, 2012). These committees have mobilized, each in its own field, to review the list of nutrients declared on the label, develop nutrient reference values and propose new claims for high-risk nutrients (*trans* fat).

However, there is an important item in the *Global Strategy* document addressed to *Codex* which refers to the modification of food production and processing standards taking into account the precepts of nutritional and health quality. The response given by the CAC was palliative in nature to protect the health of consumers, but comfortable and profitable for the market. It proposed the development of modified versions of organically unhealthy foods, differentiating them by reducing risky ingredients (salt, fats and/or sugars) in the composition and by using nutritional claims on the label, in order to help consumers distinguish and choose between these products.

From an ethical and health point of view, the specific nutritional profile proposed for modified versions of food products should be the rule, because of the added health benefits. The original food product, on the other hand, with an unhealthy profile, should be completely abolished from the market. However, it turns out that it is the economic value that stands out in this proposal (modified versions of products), due to the prospect of opening up a market for "special" food products, at a higher cost, aimed at a select public, and with a discreet impact on the health of the community. For the time being, this issue is still under discussion and has not yet gone beyond the CAC.

The *Codex* Commission's delay in getting involved with the WHO's initiatives and the proposals for intervention suggested by the WHO shows that the Commission's commitment to the health of the world's population is closely tied to the risks that impact the economic interests of the international market. This is evident when comparing the regulatory performance of the CAC against contaminants in food products with that of the delegate against excess nutrients that make products unhealthy. Risks of a different nature have little impact on the Commission, despite the visibility and global reach expressed in the epidemiological data that measures these risks.

Food products that are contaminated or that are carriers of disease circulating on the international market can have damaging intercontinental and immediate effects, both in terms of economic damage and consumer health, and in terms of boycotts of the companies involved, which can spread to other products exported from the country in which they are located. The negative effects on health caused by risks involving deviations in nutritional quality are slow to develop and last for a long time. Furthermore, they originate from highly profitable products marketed by powerful transnational corporations.

This negligent attitude towards collective demands has led to strong criticism of supranational bodies, such as the *Codex Alimentarius* Commission and the WTO, due to their current accumulation of power in the governance[16] of food systems, as they are governed by the interests of large market corporations. It is these corporations that are responsible for engendering dietary changes and disseminating their hypercaloric products globally (BRAUM, 2001; LANG, 1999). This situation has given rise to tensions and conflicts, sparking the first signs of reaction in academia (LANG, 1999; LABONTÉ; MOHINDRA; LECUCHA, 2011) and civil society (BRAUM, 2001; SANTOS, 2005).

Although the national delegations of the CAC's specific committees are made up of high-ranking government officials appointed by their governments, representatives of industry, consumer organizations and academic institutions are allowed to participate in these delegations. However, official government representatives only have the right to vote, and international organizations, including those from organized civil society, only have the right to speak (FAO; WHO, 2006b). However, depending on the interests of the government and the political pressures to which it is subjected, its vote can tend to favor the collective or private interest. This is where the legitimacy of government

---

16 Governance, at the global level, is understood as a set of intergovernmental relationships, involving non-governmental organizations (NGOs), civil movements, multinational companies and global capital markets, which bring together and articulate interests to seek solutions to common problems. The active participation of non-state actors in the scenario has contributed greatly to broadening the contributions and opinions capable of influencing results, whether in the sphere of public policy or international regulation. However, the big challenge is legitimacy, whether global society actually gives power and sees itself represented by the actors who make decisions in strategic fields on its behalf (GONÇALVES, 2005).

representatives and even organized civil society, which is not immune to such pressures, comes into question.

The economic capacity of corporations also allows them to bargain for favors and materially seduce the members of *Codex* delegations in order to meet their objectives, especially those that are weak in economic and ethical terms. It must be made clear that, in the matter in question, public interests are at odds with private ones. In this perspective, McKee's (1999) reflection points out that, since the massive participation of representatives of the production sector in *Codex* Committees, and some members of government and academia without the firmness of their commitments to the collective, the interests of consumers and citizens have been neglected.

In view of the above, emerging food risks prompt reflection and revision of the CAC's institutional conduct, so that it can effectively carry out its mission of protecting health and ensuring fair practices in the food trade.

3.1.3 The WTO and food products: profits for the market and damage to health

From 1995 onwards, the World Trade Organization (WTO)[17] , an entity that brings together 159 countries and deals with global trade rules (WTO, 2013a), adopted the standards, guidelines and recommendations established by the FAO/WHO *Codex Alimentarius* as a reference for food trade disputes. These became the legal parameters of the Agreement on the Application of Sanitary and Phytosanitary Measures - SPS Agreement (WHO/FAO, 2006). This instrument, in particular, deserves comment, as it provides for sanitary measures to protect human life and health against the risks resulting from the presence of additives and contaminants in food and drink. Although this Agreement is the result of a consensus between the member countries participating in the Organization, it limits the autonomy of national states to make their own rules in certain circumstances.

The SPS Agreement, governed by the principles of equivalence, non-discrimination, efficiency, transparency and harmonization, states that member countries are allowed to adopt or apply the necessary sanitary measures, provided that they do not constitute arbitrary or unjustifiable discrimination and are based on scientific principles. Preferably in line with the principle of harmonization, health measures should be based on

17 The WTO was created in 1994 as a result of the Uruguay Round of multilateral trade negotiations and the subsequent revision of the General Agreement on Tariffs and Trade (GATT). As a result of GATT, several agreements were approved, including the General Agreement on Sanitary and Phytosanitary Measures (SPS), which was ratified by the Brazilian government through Decree No. 1.355 of December 30, 1994.

international standards, guides and recommendations and, in the case of food risks, follow those produced by the CAC. If a country imposes health measures that are more restrictive than those approved internationally, these must be preceded by a risk assessment, in accordance with the techniques established by this body, to justify the reasons for departing from the standard. This is a highly complex and challenging procedure for many countries, should they decide to use it to justify regulating the nutritional parameters of food products.

The WTO assesses positively the most recent stage of globalization, which has resulted in increased integration of product markets and capital flows and in the dynamism of work, driven by technological innovations, increased and faster information processes. This has also been supported by the economic policies of deregulation and the facilitation of international trade, as well as the flow of international investment. According to the WTO, all this has brought important changes to many countries and their citizens. Free trade has created commercial opportunities for exporting companies that offer consumers diversified products and services at lower prices (WTO, 2008).

As for food, there has been an expansion in world food production and an increase in the profitability of production (WTO, 2008). In 2012, exports amounted to 1.375 trillion dollars, with Brazil ranking second on the list of the world's main trading countries (WTO, 2013b). Between 1990 and 2012, Brazil's food exports grew spectacularly in monetary value, from 8.697 to 77.212 million dollars (WTO, 2013c).

Despite this growing commercial success, the WTO's evaluations consider that market reform, which has made business more efficient, has culminated in the concentration of industries, the formation of international production groups and has deepened inequality, increasing unemployment and public spending. The market asymmetries reported by the WTO are almost exclusively in the economic field. This stems from an institutional vision that focuses on the market and refuses to perceive the contradictions of economic globalization as diffuse, since they also invade areas such as health and nutrition. For this reason, Rayner and colleagues (2007) state that trade policies need to go beyond quantifying the volume of production/consumption in the global food system and incorporate nutritional and dietary considerations, raising the importance of food governance for public benefit.

From another perspective, the impacts of the liberation of the international food market have been overwhelming for local food economies (PHILLIPS, 2006). Local food prices become unable to compete with those of imported foods distributed by global chains, generally unhealthy and low-cost foods, which annihilate local production, leading to a reduction in jobs and income opportunities (TULLAO, 2002). In addition, within national economies, commercial transactions carried out by large transnational agricultural and food corporations are multiplying, absorbing smaller companies. As a result, the transnationals have become even stronger, in an upward trend observed since the end of the 1990s (CHOPRA, 2002). The complex way in which these corporations operate therefore has effects on the economic, political and social spheres.

Thus, in the face of the established global order, the sovereign action of national states is hampered. They have become subject to the strong and constant influence of international food trade rules and agreements, such as those led by the WTO and *Codex*, including those dealing with quality issues and health safety standards (LUCCHESE, 2003). Furthermore, there is a constant concern on the part of those in charge of reordering the production system to influence decisions within intergovernmental organizations so as not to compromise their interests. Thus, representatives of transnational conglomerates mobilize and skillfully occupy strategic political spaces, including supranational institutions, the result of which has a direct impact on national sovereignty. According to Sklair (2002), they behave like political and economic actors who infiltrate the institutional machinery, build alliances, "engineer" research results, benefit employees, in short, mobilize various strategies and resources to make global capitalism's agenda of interests viable.

In view of this, several social scientists point out that the sovereignty of national states has been weakened by the globalization of the economy (IANNI, 2007; BECK, 1999; GIDDENS, 1991; BAUMANN, 1999); the latter now assumes the role of interlocutor of local and global politics. However, Santos (2005) states that the state is still strong, despite the power of transnational companies and supranational institutions, because they do not have the regulatory power alone to impose their political and economic will on a particular country. Even if it is controversial, this global-local dominance makes it difficult to develop market control policies that suit the particular social interests of each national space, as it masks diversity and social and cultural specificity (MALUF; VALENTE; MENEZES, 1996), as well as tending to privilege private economic interests over collective demands.

In recent years, there has been an intellectual uprising by independent professionals and consumer groups who, although they have not yet achieved sufficient expressiveness to contain the direction of these institutions and organizations (SKLAIR, 2002), are spreading their dissatisfaction and forming opinions. From the point of view of government and civil society, isolated reactions are beginning to emerge in some countries (PUSKA, 2004; HAWKES, 2007; BRASIL; MS, 2012). However, there is still a long way to go before the issue of "improving food quality" is consolidated on the platform of public health struggles.

In the case of the Brazilian government, in addition to formal links with these international organizations, there are also links with the Southern Common Market[18] - Mercosur, which involves agreements that include health requirements. Within Mercosur, health issues are dealt with in the Working Subgroup⁰ 11, created with GMC Resolution⁰ 151/96, which has the task of harmonizing the laws of the States Parties with regard to goods, services, raw materials and products in the health area, as well as the criteria for epidemiological surveillance. It also seeks to make health control systems compatible in order to promote and protect people's health and lives and to eliminate obstacles to regional trade (BRASIL; MS, 2007a). In the case of food products, the *Codex Alimentarius* standards prevail in discussions (QUEIROZ; GIOVANELLA, 2011) and so the issue of the nutritional quality of food products still remains distant from this economic bloc.

This world of interconnected economic and social relations is part of the context in which food products are discussed, which prevents them from being treated as objects confined to national space. Since the risks of globalized food make private world trade profitable, improving the parameters of food requires a great deal of effort, including the mobilization of resources and various links, both nationally and internationally. This is politically exhausting, but essential if we are to protect the health of our communities.

3.2 Globalization of food products: health at stake

3.2.1 *Advances and setbacks in the food market*

Driven by globalization, the food market has expanded the availability and diversity of products, even without simultaneously providing universal access to them. As a result, it

18 Mercosur is an economic bloc made up of the member states Argentina, Brazil, Paraguay, Uruguay and Venezuela. It was created on March 26, 1991, by a Constitutive Charter - the Treaty of Assunçâo. With the signing of the Treaty of Ouro Preto in 1994, it was given national and international legal personality. It is based on the free movement of goods, services and productive factors, and reciprocity of rights and obligations between the States Parties (BRASIL; MS, 2007a). The Common Market Council is the highest political body, followed by the Mercosur General Group, which also acts as the bloc's decision-making body (BRASIL; MS, 2003).

has profoundly interfered with food culture, dietary consumption patterns and the nutritional status of many of the world's populations (KENNEDY; NANTEL; SHETTY, 2006). In this expansion process, the market has been improved by technological advances, especially in the field of fat chemistry (DREWNOWSKI, 2003), changes in the price of vegetable oils (WHO, 2003b), the discovery of new sources of sugar - originating from corn and at a lower cost (BEGHIN; JENSEN, 2008), as well as modern marketing techniques (HAWKES, 2002). Supported by international investment, this market has made the competition between globally circulated food products and nationally sourced food more fierce, in terms of price, availability and other commercial attributes, which has led to the gradual replacement of local food agents by global ones.

This set of innovations was an important driver of changes in dietary preferences, with the introduction of unhealthy, low-cost industrialized foods, as well as in the nutrition and health of a significant contingent of people (UUSITALO, PIETIENEN & PUSKA, 2002). In the second half of the 20th century, these changes led to the emergence of the new risks of the contemporary era in industrialized regions and, subsequently, in developing countries (WHO, 2003b).

During the consolidation of this new type of food product on the market, from the mid-1960s to the last years of the 1990s, two phenomena in opposite directions marked the changes in dietary patterns: an increase in the availability of calories worldwide of around 450 kilocalories (Kcal) *per capita per* day, exceeding 600 Kcal in developing countries; and a decline in the consumption of basic products - roots, tubers and cereals - and fruit and vegetables, accompanied by an increase in vegetable oils and meat products, excluding fish, and an increase in the proportion of energy from added sugars in diets (WHO, 2003b).

It's important to note that the first phenomenon mentioned made it possible to increase the caloric intake of the diet of parts of the population that were surviving on limited food consumption. In the 1970s, there was a scenario of poverty and disease in the world, in which the number of children dying between the ages of zero and five was almost double - 17 million - what is estimated today. This situation was strictly linked to the extreme poverty of these children (WHO, 2003c).

From the perspective of Mazzocchi, Shankar & Traill (2012), these dietary changes occurred in two stages: the first resulted in the 'expansion effect', with an increase in the energy supply from cheaper food products of plant origin, while respecting culture, beliefs and religious traditions. In the second, there was the 'substitution effect', a change in the consumption of food products - without a change in the total energy supply - which corresponded to the substitution of complex carbohydrates (cereals, roots and tubers) for vegetable oils, animal products (dairy and meat foods) and sugar. These changes can either indicate an improvement (if there is an increase in fruit and vegetables) or a detriment to the diet (if there is an increase in sugar and saturated fat).

In almost all Latin American countries, between 1990 and 1999, there was an increase in energy availability, except in Venezuela. In the mid-1990s, consumption of cereals, roots, fruit and vegetables declined slightly, while that of animal protein (meat, fish, eggs, milk and dairy products), sugar and fats increased. The traditional Latin American dietary pattern, rich in complex polysaccharides, micronutrients and fibre, is beginning to be reconfigured, with the inclusion of high quantities of refined sugars, animal products and highly processed foods, due to the impacts of the globalization of the diet (BERMUDEZ & TUCKER, 2003).

Meanwhile, the invasion of food products continues and extends to extreme territories. As the market in high-income countries is depleted, new bases for food corporations have been driven by the increase in the average global income spent on food, as evidenced in developing countries (MOODIE et al, 2013). They are thus mobilizing to attract new consumers and expand their sales to these new markets. With a narrow focus on making extraordinary profits, these corporations sell their food products, invented with technologies that use low-cost mixtures of ingredients and high levels of sugar, fat, salt and additives, with the support of a robust advertising apparatus (CHOPRA, 2002; MOODIE et al, 2013; HAWKES, 2002; MONTEIRO, 2009). They enter these countries completely free and without any ethical commitments to offer their products, which do little to nourish, but have many effects on the health of the population (STUCKLER & NESTLE, 2012).

In many of these countries, the entry of transnational food corporations has been encouraged by different mechanisms, some of which have already been discussed in this paper. These are: foreign direct investment in the food production chain, the reduction of barriers, and the control and pressure exerted on local agricultural production. These mechanisms both reduce the price of raw materials and disrupt local markets. This creates a political and economic environment that creates a market for highly processed products, to the detriment of healthy food and local culture, as well as other harmful effects on the health and economy of the countries where these companies are established (LABONTÉ; MOHINDRA; LECUCHA, 2011).

As a result, there have been changes in the profile of Asian - Chinese and Japanese - diets, which were previously rich in complex carbohydrates, and in Brazilian diets, as a result of the probable connection between innate sensory preferences, the greater availability of cheap fats in the global economy and rapid social changes in low-income societies (DREWNOWSKI; POPKIN, 1997). A similar phenomenon is also occurring in India (VEPA, 2006). In this context, it is possible to infer that, for the poor in these societies, gaining access to food is only one stage. There are still other challenges to be faced in order to bridge the gap between accessibility and the guarantee of a nutritionally healthy product.

In Central America, the reduction in import tariffs on food products from the United States resulted in changes to the usual diet, the inhibition of local production and an increase in food imports, which rose by 115% between the beginning of the 1990s and the new millennium. Alongside the increase in the availability of meat, fruit and vegetables - a promising effect - there has also been an increase in ultra-processed products (sweets, *cookies*, *crisps*, snacks and the like), associated with the nutritional transition and implications for diseases (THOW; HAWKES, 2009).

In short, traditional eating habits and practices are falling apart in different parts of the world, both in little-known places such as Tonga in Oceania (EVANS et al, 2001) and in strategic locations such as Brazil, where traditional foods in the national diet - such as beans, manioc flour, rice and corn flour - are being consumed less and less and are gradually being replaced by ultra-processed products, especially in extra-home meals (BEZERRA et al, 2013). Data from the most recent Family Budget Survey (POF 2008-2009) revealed that the lowest-income urban families in Brazil invest proportionally more money in soft drinks, cookies and pasta than the highest-income families (BRASIL; IBGE, 2011). According to Bleil (1998), all of these changes in diet occur with the support of the advertising structure, which imposes global culture as a symbol of modernity, conceals market interests, destroys local culture and omits the risks of the products on offer.

The mechanisms used don't even spare the traditional Mediterranean diet, recognized worldwide for its legitimate reputation for being healthy. The results of the latest national survey reveal that Spanish students are replacing conventional foods with unhealthy industrialized foods, such as pasta, soft drinks, fruit juices, cakes, *snacks* and *fast food*; and rejecting leafy greens, vegetables and fish (FERNANDEZ SAN JUAN, 2006). However, this is not unique to Spain, as the entire European population has been exposed to the harmful effects of the promotion and availability of nutritionally poor food products, especially children and adolescents from low-income backgrounds (WHO, 2006).

These transnational food corporations[19] , in addition to intervening in all stages of the production system, have a complex scheme of intercontinental movements, guided by commercial strategies, and the key business of most of them is unhealthy food products such as *snack foods*, chocolates, cereals and cookies, soft drinks and confectionery. As an illustration, the Kellogs company has processing plants in China, India, Japan, South Korea and Thailand to supply the distribution chains in Asia; Pepsico continues to expand its vast international marketing line in *snack foods*, currently focusing on Latin America and Asia-Pacific; and the Nestlé, Kraft and Unilever corporations already operate in almost 140 countries (REGMI & GEHLHAR, 2005). Nestlé, in particular, is one of the top five food companies in Brazil, India, Mexico, Russia, the United States and South Africa (MOODIE et al, 2013), which means making its products available to a contingent of people that corresponds to 27.6% of the world's population (UN, 2013).

The transnational retail trade has also benefited from rapid expansion in Latin America (LABONTÉ; MOHINDRA; LENCUCHA, 2011) and other developed countries (FAO, 2006). The United States, the European Union and Japan together dominate this type of trade and account for 60% of total retail sales of processed food products in the world (REGMI & GEHLHAR, 2005). The rapid multinationalization of supermarket chains and the way they operate are helping to consolidate a type of food consumption practice, with consequent nutritional implications. Accessibility, availability and variety are incentives to buy different food items, especially energy-dense ones. In addition, they benefit from the adoption of strategies of low prices, promotion, easy visualization and access at the point of sale that confront the unequal conditions of supply of fruit and vegetables, which tend to be more expensive due to the peculiarities of production. All of this has led to the rise in the sale of unhealthy food products, which is a significant part of the explanation for changes in habits, the increase in consumer demand and preference and chronic diseases of dietary origin (HAWKES, 2008).

The introduction of these new types of food has led to a change in the profile of food

19 They are a conglomerate of large food companies, with subsidiaries in several countries, which provide their supplies globally, centralize strategic capital, resources and decision-making and maintain operations in several countries to make the global market more unified. They behave like powerful players on the world socio-economic stage.

expenditure, the impact of which has been greater in developing countries. According to Popkin (2006), between 1990 and 2000, retail food sales in supermarkets increased by 15 to 60% in Latin America. These places sell processed and unhealthy food products, but also those of balanced nutritional quality. However, it is the products of the first type that the sales stimulus apparatus focuses on.

This increase in *per capita* spending coincides with an increase in sales of processed products in developing countries. Between 1998-2003, the countries considered to be the lowest income and lower middle income had a higher average annual growth in sales than the other countries, ranging from 8.1% to 56.3% for breakfast cereals, oils and fats, ready meals, dairy products and dry products. When these figures were compared with higher-income countries, it was observed that growth in this group of countries was minimal, with the highest rate achieved for one of these product categories being 4.7% (MAZZOCCHI; SHANKAR; TRAILL, 2012).

Although the panorama of the food market, especially the industrial and retail corporations, is brief, it is possible to understand why several studies have pointed out the interface between the globalization of the food market, the dietary transition and the international spread of risk factors for CNCDs (MOODIE et al, 2013; RAYNER et al, 2013; LABONTÉ, MOHINDRA; LECUCHA, 2011; TULLAO, 2002). As presented so far, for the internationalization of food businesses to be exceptionally successful and profitable, it was necessary to destabilize local economic life and the health of the majority of the population.

3.2.2 *Food advertising and its effects on behavior and health*

Different areas of everyday life are filled with commercial advertising for food products, aimed at different audiences, especially children. Different advertising channels and techniques are used, both conventional and current, such as television, the internet, *video games*, direct mail, posters, *billboards*, among others, which, in an insistent and continuous manner, are designed to stimulate the sale of products and, at the same time, inculcate values, habits and behaviors.

Aggressive commercial advertising of unhealthy food products, reported as symbols of social *status*, has motivated individuals, especially those living in urban and suburban areas, to substitute traditional foods (WHO, 1990). Based on evidence of the influence of advertising for *fast-food* and energy-dense, micronutrient-poor food products on the dietary choices of children and adolescents and, consequently, on the onset of overweight and obesity (WHO, 2003a), the WHO has recommended that governments regulate the trade, advertising and labeling of these products, as one of the measures to protect children from health problems related to the consumption of these foods (WHO, 2004a; WHO, 2006).

Among advertising resources, television advertising is the means of promoting products and stimulating sales that has the greatest capacity to enter homes, transform family traditions and alienate individuals, through the color, fantasies and values that are mixed with and connected to food products, creating an inseparable effect between the product and its imaginary clothing, which convinces and stimulates individuals to buy them.

Children are enticed by the persuasive power of advertising to desire products, which benefits from their inexperience and credulity (WHO, 2006). Robinson et al (2007) found that the effects of advertising affect children at an early stage of life, between 3 and 5 years of age, whose taste preferences have been associated with a leading brand in the advertising and sales of food products.

For the market, children have three characteristics that make them the biggest potential customers: the first is that they are inclined to buy all kinds of products on offer, including direct purchases with their own money; the second is their ability to influence their parents' purchasing decisions and, finally, they are the consumers of the future (SANTOS, 2009). This is the panorama that guides companies in defining the composition, image, content and means of conveying advertising materials for their food products.

According to Hastings (2006), five product categories dominate food advertising: soft drinks, pre-sweetened cereals, sweets, snacks and *fast food.* The effect of intense exposure to these types of products on children is to exacerbate excessive consumption behavior (HARRIS et al, 2009; HASTINGS et al, 2003; HAWKES, 2006). A later study, in which children were distanced from commercial television advertising for obesogenic products, concluded that such a measure could have a significant impact on reducing childhood obesity (ZIMMERMAN; BELL, 2010).

In the case of Brazil, the profile of the most advertised food products coincides with that reported by Hastings (2006). After recording 432 hours of Brazilian television on working days, between 8am and 10pm, it was observed that, of the 1,395 ads, 57.8% fell into the fats, oils, sugars and sweets group of the food pyramid, followed by the bread, cereals, rice and pasta group (21%). The dairy and meat and pulses groups reached around 10%, with a complete lack of information on fruit and vegetables (ALMEIDA;

NASCIMENTO; QUAIOTI, 2002).

In addition to the various forms of advertising that induce the consumption of food products, Chandon & Wansink (2012) also list three other elements that confer advantages on such products: the price in the short and long term; the product itself, in terms of quantity and quality, which determines how much can be consumed and, finally, the consumption environment, which includes the availability and convenience of the act of eating.

However, it can be seen that there is a sensory gear that precedes and triggers the stimulus to consume the food product. This involves different elements, such as the scenery of the advertising and the place of consumption, the visual *design of* the packaging and the practicality of consumption, the hyperpalatability, the sound produced by the crunchiness, the exuberance of the color and the oversized liquid content, which, added to the low purchase price of the product, are capable of arousing the individual's volitional act and leading them to consumption, including compulsive consumption.

With the intention of dominating the westernization of the diet movement and creating a unified world for their products, *fast food* and soft drink companies are developing worldwide, diversified and comprehensive *marketing* activities with the aim of creating new consumer habits, from adjusting prices and packaging to sponsoring sporting and philanthropic activities (HAWKES, 2002). According to this author, the Latin American region is the representative of Coca-Cola and Pepsi's first expansion experience, and today has the second highest consumption rate, surpassed only by the USA. In this region, Brazil is the country with the third highest consumption of non-alcoholic carbonated beverages - a title that does not call for celebration, but which arouses a great deal of concern given the panorama of obesity and other CNCDs in the Brazilian population.

In the United States, there is a perverse competition between *junk* food, which is the main source of revenue for food companies, and childhood obesity rates, which have been skyrocketing since the 1970s (NESTLE, 2006). According to the author, this has provoked reactions from society, which are manifested through legal action and pressure for regulation. As a result, companies have made efforts to support health programs, announce policies renouncing advertising aimed at children and make their products appear healthier by disguising them with vitamin enrichment, whole ingredients and eliminating *trans* fats. However, these companies continue to focus their advertising investments on sweets, soft drinks and snacks.

Advertising is a powerful commercial strategy for exposing a food product in order to seduce, convince and win over consumers, and also to bridge different cultures. After having experienced the phase of diversification of consumption through the increase in traditional foods, India is now facing a process of change in food culture, with the introduction of energy-dense processed foods, supported by advertising from McDonalds, Coca-Cola, Pepsi and the like, and by *fast-food* and supermarket chains (PINGALI; KHWAJA, 2004). These changes had multiple economic and social effects, such as sudden adjustments in the local production chain to meet the demands of foreign corporations, as well as accelerated changes in the health profile and rates of chronic diseases in the country's urban centers.

Although there are some knowledge gaps to confirm the advertising-high consumption of unhealthy products-obesity triad (McDERMOTT; STEAD; HASTINGS, 2007) and the concrete impact of advertising regulation on childhood obesity prevention (HAWKES, 2007), several authors advocate the control of food advertising to children (McDERMOTT; STEAD; HASTINGS, 2007; HAWKES, 2007; NESTLE, 2006; STUCKLER; NESTLE, 2012; WHO, 2006) and countries are beginning to institute specific compulsory rules (HAWKES, 2006).

As advertising does not dispense with school environments, as they are ideal places to reach children and adolescents, control instruments are being put in place to avoid negative impacts on their health. Thus, regulations governing the consumption of food in these establishments have been approved in countries such as Brazil, France and the United States. When there are obstacles to defining regulatory rules, guidelines are established on the subject, as has happened in Fiji, the United Kingdom and Canada (HAWKES, 2007).

There is undoubtedly a link between the advertising and marketing of unhealthy food products and health risks, which has put the ethical conduct of food companies under suspicion. This is expressed in different ways: by failing to encourage individuals, especially children, to make choices favorable to the care and maintenance of their health (HAWKES, 2007) and by placing on people and society the sole burden of carrying the burden of disease induced by systematic market stimuli. This kind of disregard for ethics goes against rights in two respects - the protection of children and the preservation of health. Public intervention in the field of advertising regulation is therefore fully justified in order to protect these rights, which are threatened by unbridled commercial activity.

3.2.3 *Palatability, satiety, cost and practicality of food products*

A number of studies are trying to uncover the mechanisms that trigger the stimuli that lead to excessive consumption of unhealthy foods and have an impact on obesity and CNCD rates. Two characteristics of these foods have been selected for investigation: palatability and satiety. The former because it enhances the pleasure of tasting and the latter because of its relationship between energy cost and satisfaction.

During the investigation, it was found that palatability and satiety, related to appetite and satisfaction of consumption respectively, produce interdependent effects. In unhealthy food products, the behavior of these effects is the opposite: increasing consumption reduces the speed of the satiety response; *in fresh* foods, increasing consumption gradually leads to satiety (SWINBURN et al, 2004; DREWNOWSKI, 1999).

This inverse effect mechanism is explained by the fact that the satiety index is inversely proportional to the availability of energy and directly proportional to the weight of the food consumed, which means that foods with diluted energy tend to be more satiating but less palatable, while energy-dense foods are more palatable and less satiating (DREWNOWSKI et al, 2004).

Energy density, nutritional composition, volume and sensory aspects differentiate palatable foods from satiating foods. In the first group, the high content of sugar, fat and energy, together with low volume and sweet and fatty aspects, form its framework (potato chips, cookies, etc.), while the opposite characteristics form the profile of foods with high satiety power (fruit, vegetables, etc.). In short, foods with a high energy density that contain sugar and fat are more palatable and less satiating (DREWNOWSKI, 1999).

Swinburn and colleagues (2004) explain how fatty and sweet foods behave in terms of palatability and satiety. High-fat foods have a weak impact on satiety because the fat carries aromatic compounds that flavor the food, making it highly palatable and, in part, leading to uncontrolled overconsumption. Thus, the high palatability, coupled with the relatively weak metabolic self-regulation of high-fat diets, is the challenge. As for the sugar content, the author states that although it seems to limit the hedonic response, sweetness also increases the palatability of many foods, which also seems to lead to overconsumption. In this sense, since fat and sugar are linked to increasing the palatability of food, processed products with a high content of these two components can lead to weight gain. When the author refers to the energy intake of beverages, such as soft drinks, he says that it is low because it is diluted by the high water content in these products. The same author argues that, in physiological terms, the impact of the energy density of solid foods cannot be transposed to liquid foods, and it is prudent to consider it separately.

Another relevant point relates to the monetary cost of food in relation to its energy density, which is extremely important to consider when designing public nutrition policies, because it has a direct impact on the budget of low-income families. DREWNOWSKI (2010) states that foods considered healthy, such as vegetables, fruit and meat, poultry and fish, have an extremely high monetary cost per calorie and higher levels of protein, minerals and vitamin C, compared to sugars, sweets and beverages and oils, fats and sauces. However, the fruit and vegetable groups had the lowest energy density and exceeded the other groups in water content and cost of the average portion served, making them more expensive in terms of energy cost compared to the whole group analyzed. In another study, Andrieu, Darmon & Drewnowski (2006), using records of French diets, reconfirmed that free choice low cost diets tend to be energy dense and poor in key nutrients, except for calcium and fiber. Antioxidant vitamins, present in fruit and vegetables, were associated with a higher energy cost.

Food products with high palatability, high energy density, built-in social value and relatively low cost are elements that attract consumers, despite being considered "unhealthy". There is also the practicality of consuming them, as most of the time they are ready-made or require minimal heating, which is important in a daily life where time is of the essence.

Finally, food products with high palatability and low satiety power are the success of transnational food companies, whose global spread has interfered in the lives, health and economy of many populations, regardless of their position in the life cycle, with the poor being the most affected, as will be shown in the following chapter.

4 THE DYNAMICS OF TRANSITIONS: DIETETICS, NUTRITION AND EPIDEMIOLOGY

4.1 The journey from the dietary transition to the nutritional transition

During the bibliographical survey, the use of the term "*dietary transition*" (WHO, 1990) was changed to "*nutritional transition*" (WHO, 2002b) in official WHO documents, and in other scientific articles (CHOPRA, 2002, POPKIN, 2006), both of which establish distinct parallels with transformations in the nutritional and epidemiological profile of populations. In this sense, brief considerations will be made about the context used and its implications for understanding nutritional phenomena.

In 1990, the WHO used the *dietary transition* to explain the changes that had taken place in diet over the previous four decades, arguing that they had resulted in an increase in the consumption of saturated fats, simple carbohydrates, smoked and salt-preserved *foods, snack foods*, alcoholic drinks, *pickles* and a decrease in the consumption of vegetables and fruit, the effects of which had repercussions on the pattern of morbidity and mortality, increasing the rates of obesity, coronary heart disease, diabetes, hypertension, cancer, etc. (WHO, 1990). The *dietary transition*, then, is situated in the body of transformations that have taken place in the composition of the diet, and is explained by a set of elements that show changes in the types of nutrients and foods that are harmful to health. Diet is assumed to be one of the factors related to changes in the type and frequency of diseases.

The dietary transition is analyzed as a specific phenomenon that has taken place in parallel with changes in lifestyle, which have led to a reduction in physical activity and an increase in stress, among other factors, which have changed the pattern of morbidity and mortality. These were changes of various kinds, occurring over the same period of time, and transforming the disease profile of emerging countries, bringing it into line with that of affluent countries. One of these changes occurred in the dietary pattern.

In this context, diet and lifestyle are presented as associated entities, but they are not properly articulated to allow them to be observed as events that interact with each other and lead to an increase or decrease in the conditions of exposure to the risk of disease.

About a decade later, the WHO adopted the term *nutritional transition* to summarize the changes in risk factors and diseases. This is the increase in the consumption of high-calorie processed products (rich in sugars and low-cost fats) to the detriment of raw foods, in a context of reduced physical activity, which is contributing to the obesity epidemic and the increase in the prevalence of other CNCDs, and which is coexisting with residual malnutrition (WHO, 2002b). The WHO goes on to explain that the rising levels of NCDs are due to changes in diet, in terms of quality and quantity, and physical inactivity, linked to inadequate work and leisure patterns. It also points out that this experience is now manifesting itself especially in developing countries (WHO, 2003b).

This transition therefore marks the confrontation of developing countries with two nutrition phenomena, of apparently opposite natures, but with a common essential feature: on the one hand, the emerging challenge of overweight, obesity and other NCDs and, on the other, the permanence of undernourishment and micronutrient deficiencies in the population. However, these two nutritional problems have combined and concentrated on poor social strata in these groups of countries.

It can be seen that in the "*nutritional transition*", there is no dissociation between the transitions in diet, diseases and physical activity behaviors. They are all interconnected in this concept. This concept also uses the generic term "diet", but there is the addition of another specific term, which names and qualifies the foods involved: low-cost, high-calorie industrialized products.

The understanding of the *nutritional transition* has improved and it has come to be seen as a process that reveals an inversion in the patterns of distribution of nutritional problems in a given population over time, being referenced by the rise in the prevalence of obesity and the rapid decline in malnutrition (BATISTA FILHO; RISSIN, 2003), and is linked to different stages of the country's economic and social development (KAC; VELÀSQUEZ-MELÉNDEZ, 2003).

In view of the above, it can be seen that the *nutritional transition* is beginning to break away from a strictly technical approach, devoid of any mention of political and economic components, and is now being recognized as an event specific to the dynamics of society and, therefore, derived from the social transformations that have revolutionized global nutrition, especially food consumption practices.

In Brazil, the *nutritional transition* was consolidated very quickly, in just three decades, as shown by the results of three national surveys: the National Study on Family Expenditure (ENDEF)-1974/75; the National Health and Nutrition Survey (PNSN)-1989; and the National Demographic and Health Survey (PNDS)-1995/96 (BATISTA FILHO; RISSIN, 2003). However, in the 2002/03 POF, there was still a decline in the prevalence of underweight by age in children under five, reaching 4.6% - when compared to the result of 16.6% obtained in the 1974/75 ENDEF - and, at the same time, an increase in obesity and overweight in adults (COUTINHO; GENTIL; TORAL, 2008). According to these authors, the inversion of nutritional standards was a reflection of the influence of the intense transformations that took place in Brazilian society, which gave a positive boost to the living conditions of the poorest strata, including facilitating access to food, which does not necessarily indicate an increase in the consumption of foods with an adequate nutritional profile.

Popkin's (2002) article decoded the *nutritional transition* in developing countries in more detail and his analysis brought it closer to current socio-economic events. According to this author, the *nutritional transition* is an integral part of the context of the rapid globalization of the food market, communication systems, urbanization and individual lifestyles. This has interfered with changes in the general structure of dietary patterns and encouraged a sedentary lifestyle over the last two decades. Evidence closely associated with the demographic and epidemiological transition, characterized by changes in the average height, body composition and morbidity of populations. A little later, Popkin & Gordon-Larsen (2004) focused on exploring the dietary changes that occurred during this transition separately.

Over the years, the *nutritional transition,* as well as the growth of NCDs, have come to be understood as immediate results of the globalization of the human diet (UUSITALO, PIETNEN & PUSKA, 2002; WHO, 2003b), and therefore as one of the negative effects of economic globalization (WHO, 2005). Economic growth, the transformation of the food system and the *nutritional transition* are synchronized and dependent events (FAO, 2013b). This brings to light important players in this phenomenon, whose behavior contributes to the *nutritional transition*. They are: the market, through its domination of the trade in unhealthy food products and intensive advertising, which destroys healthy eating patterns, and food regulators, through their inertia in intervening in the excessive behavior of the market, which deteriorates the nutritional quality of products.

In short, the *dietary transition* is a facet of the *nutritional transition*, which in turn is part of the social transition. The translation of this phenomenon is not limited to changes in diet or the predominance of obesity compared to malnutrition. It is a complex social phenomenon which, in the debate over the years, has come to be understood as the result of the impacts of economic and social relations in the global sphere, reflected in the field of human nutrition.

4.2 Obesity and other NCDs on the rise: global and national panorama

4.2.1 *Obesity and its comorbidities around the world: brief comments*

The changes imposed on society as a result of the process of economic globalization have diversified health risks. In this context, food is one of the factors involved, creating new types of illness, without however eliminating the traditional events that lead to poor nutrition or food-borne illnesses. This gives rise to a picture of nutritional diseases marked by the consumption of food involving specific aspects - or their intersections - such as reduced or excessive quantity, inadequate nutritional and/or health quality. However, in this work, the approach will be restricted to the adverse effects of consuming food with inadequate nutritional quality.

At the end of the 20th century, the WHO proclaimed obesity to be a global epidemic (WHO, 2000), which originated in the United States, spread to Europe and other wealthy nations in the world and gradually reached the countries of the transition economies, until it ended its worldwide circuit in the countries considered to be poor (PRENTICE, 2005; WHO, 2000). It is a type of chronic disease that has spread to all continents and has the peculiarity of affecting individuals from different age groups and social strata. This makes for a complex epidemiological picture that mobilizes huge public resources, both for the treatment of the disease in question and the related comorbidities (WHO, 2000, CABALLERO, 2007). The rising prevalence of obesity and its complications has become a major threat to public health worldwide (WHO, 2000; VISSCHER & SEIDELL, 2001).

According to the WHO, the close relationship between energy-dense diets and sedentary lifestyles has contributed to the rise of a list of CNCDs - obesity, diabetes mellitus, cardiovascular diseases, hypertension, heart attacks and some types of cancer - which are becoming major causes of premature death and disability in developing and developed countries (WHO, 2003b). Between the 1970s and 1980s, there was a 105% relative increase in chronic diseases in tropical South America, at a time when changes in lifestyle and diet were taking place. In this context, food emerged as one of the main modifiable determinants of this type of disease (WHO, 1990).

In 2005, out of a total of 58 million deaths, 35 million (60%) were the result of NCDs. In 2008, this global estimate rose to 36 million out of a total of 57 million deaths (UN, 2013). The main modifiable risk factors for this group of diseases are an unhealthy diet, physical inactivity and smoking (WHO, 2005); alcohol consumption is not included in the list of these factors.

In 2012, NCDs continue to be one of the main public health challenges and remain at 60% of global deaths, threatening economic and social development and requiring a concerted effort at local level. As a result, many countries are already developing various fronts to prevent and control these diseases by intervening in risk factors such as unhealthy diet, physical inactivity and overweight and obesity (WHO, 2013a).

As a chronic morbidity, obesity stands out in the group of CNCDs because it is capable, in isolation, of triggering multiple morbid events such as type II diabetes mellitus, cardiovascular disease, osteoarthritis, cancer and respiratory disorders, as well as psychosocial problems such as incapacity for work, low self-esteem and others (WHO, 2004a; UUSITALO; PIETIENEN; PUSKA, 2002; VISSCHER; SEIDELLL, 2001; WHO, 2000). Although there is no age limit for the onset of obesity and it can be detected early in life, the age at which the disease begins and its degree of severity will signal the persistence of this disease and its deleterious effects throughout adulthood (MUST, 1996). Among the critical periods for the development of obesity are the prenatal period, the period of adipose repletion between five and seven years of age and the period of adolescence (DIETZ, 1994), which require special attention in view of the future implications.

On the European continent, overweight is a growing health problem. The prevalence of overweight fluctuated between 32% and 79% among men and between 28% and 78% among women, while the prevalence of obesity was narrower: between 5%-23% and 7%-36%, respectively, for men and women, according to data obtained between 1999 and 2005 (BRANCA; NIKOGOSIAN; LOBSTEIN, 2007). However, according to these authors, both disorders contribute to 80% of cases of type II diabetes, 35% of ischemic heart disease and 55% of hypertension in adults. In Spain, specifically, in the period 1987-1997, there was a 71% relative increase in the prevalence of obesity in adult men and 63% in adult women: the biggest increases occurred in the adult population with no schooling, in both sexes, according to the results of national surveys (GUTIÉRREZ-FISAC et al, 2003).

Although Africa is low on cases of malnutrition, obesity is already present in the north-east, particularly in Morocco and Tunisia (MOKHTAR et al, 2001), as well as in other countries on the continent (WHO, 2004a; WHO, 2005). In Asia's most populous country - China - obesity already affects more than 20% of children and adolescents aged between 7 and 17 living in urban centers (WHO, 2005).

In a group of 17 Latin American countries analyzed, AMIGO (2003) found an average prevalence of obesity close to 4.5% in children under five years of age, and in four of them the figures were higher than 6%, indicating that there are increases in rates, although they are still not considered high. Obesity among Latin American women in nine countries in the region was on the rise during the 1990s, with rates ranging from 7.6 to 12.1%, except in Haiti (KAIN; VIO; ALBALA, 2003). Between 1990 and 2010, the estimate of combined overweight and obesity among children of the same age in this part of the world rose from 4% to 7% (MEERMAN; CARISMA; THOMPSON, 2012).

The main chronic diseases that contribute to premature deaths are related to lifestyle risk factors - excessive consumption of unhealthy products, smoking and alcohol, as well as physical inactivity.

According to the WHO (WHO, 2004a), these are recognized as global diseases, with a preventive nature; however, the explanation given for their causality presents misconceptions, such as individual culpability, social and age restrictions, as well as a preponderantly genetic susceptibility. These facts have covered up the responsibilities to be assumed by governments and industries, social vulnerability to disease, the interaction of social and not exclusively genetic risk factors and the collective damage caused by the failure to adopt public control and prevention measures.

Individual responsibility requires special consideration. This is because the "new public health", guided by neoliberal principles, advocates that the solution lies with individuals, as citizens who are free and competent to exercise self-control, define their lifestyles and make choices that protect their health, disregarding the importance of structural determinants (PETERSON; LUPTON, 2000), where health problems really originate. Tanaka & Nakanishi (1996), addressing the growth of NCDs in Japan at the end of the 20th century, based precisely on this neoliberal idea, point out that individuals can reduce or eliminate risk factors for cardiovascular diseases, except for factors such as age, heredity and gender, by modifying certain lifestyle choices, such as diet, physical exercise, stress, smoking and alcohol.

It's essential to reflect on these issues, because blaming the individual alone for the fate of their health, particularly because they don't have the skills to move their body enough or know how to select food or restrain themselves from consuming stimuli, is a simplistic analysis for effectively dealing with the causal complexity of NCDs. There is a global phenomenon of diseases that necessarily has a common root. Understanding it implies recovering the underlying and essential social elements that are the basis of the causal determination process. It is then a question of deciphering the relationships between individual societies and the context of the global economy aimed at mass consumption, the weakness of public institutions to intervene in the private world, the weakness of social movements to demand and become aware of collective morbid phenomena, etc.

It should be noted that individuals, in the sphere of the consumer goods market in contemporary society, are almost undone beings, because, according to Bauman (2008), their virtues have been weakened, their condition as thinking and autonomous subjects has been erased, making them incapable of consciously reflecting and deciding on the goods on offer. Individuals have become mere potential objects of consumption, constantly being deceived, seduced and maneuvered by powerful pressures from private businesses. These conditions have also made it difficult for individuals to properly select the food they eat in order to protect their own health.

Thus, to place the responsibility on the individual to contain the risks and therefore to promote health and prevent disease, is to artificially force the exclusion of the strategic players in the scenario - the public authorities and the economic sectors - especially those that produce industrialized foods.

4.2.2 The Brazilian epidemiological picture and its connection with the world's ills

The portrait of the Brazilian epidemiological profile clearly shows the global marks of the process of internationalization of food production, which insistently strives to homogenize the consumption practices and behaviour of the planet. All this to make it possible to concentrate the wealth that feeds back into its dynamism, with the effects being chronic ills - disease and poverty - that are socialized with the majority of the population.

In Brazil, the recent picture of the main chronic diseases in the adult population points to 22.7% suffering from hypertension, 5.6% from diabetes and 15.8% from obesity, and 48.5% of individuals are already overweight (BRASIL; MS,

2012b). These diseases have shown increasing rates of prevalence since 2006 (SCHMIDT et al, 2011; BRASIL; MS, 2012b).

According to these authors, of the total number of deaths recorded in 2007, around 72% were attributed to NCDs; the explanatory panorama for the increase in exposure to this group of diseases includes improved access to food and the globalization of unhealthy eating habits. It is precisely the lack of communication between easier access to food and its nutritional quality that leads to the emergence of risks and chronic diseases.

Previous national surveys, PNAD-2003 and PNAD-2008, indicate that the increase in hypertension and diabetes and the higher prevalence of most chronic diseases, with the exception of tendinitis/tenosynovitis and cancer, are concentrated in the segments of the population with less schooling and without private health insurance benefits. In the opinion of these authors, this evidence expresses the social inequalities in the manifestation of this group of diseases, a situation that is also observed in other countries (BARROS et al, 2011). Another study showed something similar when it analyzed the behavior of risk factors in the population, such as altered blood pressure levels, obesity and excessive alcohol consumption, which were also associated with groups with worse living conditions (OLIVEIRA-CAMPOS, RODRIGUES-NETO, SILVEIRA, NEVES et al, 2013).

Chronic diseases, like any other manifestation of the health-disease process, are socially shaped. It is the 'social' that defines the degree of exposure to risk factors, biological susceptibility to certain diseases, resistance, the capacity for prevention and reaction, as well as the speed of aggravation, sequelae and death.

Considering the important role that obesity plays as a precursor to other CNCDs (WHO, 2004), it is worth exploring the characteristics of obesity in Brazil, in terms of age and social distribution, as well as its interrelationship with the food consumed and physical activity.

The process of increasing overweight and obesity has taken place over the last three decades and has been confirmed by national surveys (BATISTA FILHO; RISSIN, 2003), as already mentioned in this paper. In the last national POF survey 20082009, the prevalence of overweight and obesity in adolescents (10 to 19 years old) was 20.5% and 4.9%, respectively, which reinforces the predisposition to the disease at a young age. In adulthood, the prevalence of obesity among men and women was 12.5% and 16.9%, respectively; the highest frequencies of overweight and obesity were in the 45-54 age groups among men and 55-64 among women, declining in subsequent age groups (BRASIL; IBGE, 2010). This progressive increase in obesity is already recognized as an emerging health problem in the Brazilian population and, together with persistent deficiency diseases, was incorporated into the government's political agenda at the end of the 1990s, becoming one of the intervention objectives of the National Food and Nutrition Policy - PNAN (BRASIL; MS, 1999).

Overweight indicators are dynamic in nature, suffering from the effects of social mobility and differing between the sexes and levels of formal education. From the 1990s onwards, the prevalence of overweight, previously concentrated in the richest regions, shifted to the poorest regions of the country and to the poorest income strata (MONDINI; MONTEIRO, 1998), while there was a stabilization in the upward trend of the problem among adult women with higher incomes (BATISTA FILHO; RISSIN, 2003).

A similar effect occurs when the social marker of schooling is used; initially, the risk of obesity covered all adults and, from that moment on, the increase occurred in individuals with low schooling, stabilizing or even decreasing in those with medium and high schooling (MONTEIRO; CONDE; CASTRO, 2003). The frequency of overweight and obesity increased in both men and women, and the average increase was higher in women in both cases. However, it can be seen that these events behave differently when they are related to the level of schooling: in the male group, the highest rates are in the stratum with the most schooling, while among women, the highest rates are in the stratum with the least schooling (BRASIL; IBGE, 2010).

More recent data indicate that overweight and obesity in adults living in the 27 Brazilian capitals and the Federal District persisted as public health problems, indicating signs of a positive trend during the last six years of monitoring the Vigitel System[20] , with rates equivalent to 48.5% and 15.8%, respectively, in 2011 (BRASIL; MS, 2012b). The two most recent Vigitel surveys, 2012 and 2013, found that the obesity rate in adults had practically stabilized, standing at 17.4% and 17.5%, respectively, while overweight was reduced from 50.8% in 2012 to 45.35% in 2013 (BRASIL; MS, 2013; BRASIL; MS, 2014).

Annually updated information on diet and physical activity is also part of the Vigitel system's data collection. The results of this survey, in 2010, revealed that only 30% of those interviewed consumed five or more portions of fruit and vegetables a week; 34% consumed excessively fatty meat; 30% practiced physical activity during leisure time or on the way to work and 28% watched three or more hours of television a day (DUNCAN; CHOR; AQUINO, 2012). In 2011, fruit and vegetable consumption among this population fell to 20.2% and the other indicators remained practically stable (BRASIL; MS, 2012b). The data for 2013 shows an increase in fruit and vegetable consumption (36%) and in physical activity (49%), a slight decrease in the consumption of fatty meat (31%) and stable behavior in time spent watching television (28.6%), in all cases maintaining the

20 Vigitel System - Surveillance of risk and protective factors for chronic diseases by telephone survey - instituted by the Ministry of Health in 2006, with the aim of monitoring the frequency and distribution of the main determinants of chronic non-communicable diseases (CNCD) in the population aged 18 or over, by telephone survey, in all the capitals of the 26 Brazilian states and the Federal District.

same specifications of the aforementioned indicators.

These lifestyle characteristics - based on sedentary lifestyles (physical inactivity) and/or the consumption of products considered unhealthy (fatty meat), are risk factors for the acquisition of chronic diseases. Thus, it is on the basis of this combination of factors that favor the onset of obesity that various authors have started to refer to the concept of an "obesogenic" environment (EGGER; SWINBURN, 1997; WHO, 2004a; CHOPRA; GALBRAITH; DARNTON-HILL, 2002; PRENTICE, 2005, CABALLERO, 2007). However, a comparative analysis of the results of the Vigitel system in recent years points to a slight trend towards a change in the nutritional profile of adults, which may signify adherence to a conduct consistent with a healthier life.

This health problem is not confined to adulthood. Overweight began to affect children at the end of the 1990s, when the prevalence rate of overweight in children aged 6 to 9 more than tripled between the two national surveys - ENDEF 1975 and the Pesquisa sobre Padrões de Vida -PPV[21] -1996-7 - rising from 4.9% to 17.4% (COSTA; CINTRA; FISBERG, 2006), and also extending to adolescence (TERRES et al, 2006; VASCONCELOS; SILVA, 2003). Different factors, such as the degree of intensity of physical activity and the mother's biotype, influence the body weight of adolescents (BURBANO; FORNASINI; ACOSTA, 2003), inadequate eating habits (NOBRE et al, 2006) and high socioeconomic status (RONQUE et al, 2005).

Despite the importance of NCDs in the national morbidity picture, the typical diseases of poverty have not been completely extinguished; and what in another historical context was referred to as the disease of opulence - obesity - is now pandemic and chronic. Because of the association between food consumption and morbid effects, the intergovernmental institutions FAO and WHO began to treat obesity as one of the manifestations of poor nutrition. With this, the term "malnutrition" became all-encompassing and came to encompass all forms of inadequate and persistent dietary intake, resulting in underweight, micronutrient deficiencies, as well as overweight and obesity.

The paradoxical coexistence of adult obesity and childhood malnutrition has been documented in Central and South American countries (PRENTICE, 2005) and other developing economies (POPKIN, 2001; WHO, 2000), including Brazil (DOAK et al, 2000;

21 This latest national survey was limited, as it only looked at the Northeast and Southeast regions of the country.

RODRIGUES, TADDEI & SEGULEM, 1998). This double and contradictory biological-social phenomenon - malnutrition and obesity - serves to reinforce the link of subordination between the exposure of individuals to nutritional diseases and poor living conditions. The link between poverty and obesity is made through access to inadequate nutritional food and sedentary leisure time (MARINHO et al, 2003), or even as a result of previous malnutrition in adult women and the short stature of children living in adverse environments (MARTINS et al, 2007). In conditions of poverty, healthy eating for obese women becomes a luxury, given the incompatibility between the high price of healthy foods (e.g. fruit and vegetables) and the income earned (FERREIRA et al, 2010).

Certainly, this approach shapes a picture of nutritional changes that is not restricted to a medical issue; rather, it is the effect of the social (dis)order that is expressed in poverty, nutritional disorders and discrimination (MEERMAN; CARISMA; THOMPSON, 2012; FAO, 2013b; WHO, 2000), signaling the decisive role of governments in tackling the complexity of this phenomenon, which requires the design and implementation of articulated and comprehensive public policies, with the aim of addressing the inequities present within society.

Thus, considering the extreme importance of food products in the etiology of obesity and other CNCDs (CHOPRA, 2002), the focus of governments should be on prevention and control. It is necessary to guide people in the field of food and nutrition and to intervene in the food production chain, both to encourage and subsidize healthy foods and to discipline those considered to be high in calories and low in nutrition. Although these are relevant and urgent measures, other strategies aimed at improving material living conditions deserve to be combined with them.

5 FOOD REGULATION: THE CHALLENGE OF GOVERNING THE MARKET

5.1 From the military regime to the democratic rule of law: the evolution of food regulation devices

In recent decades, the term "regulation" has become more popular and has spread from the economic to the administrative and social fields. However, food health regulation, in the broad sense, is a practice that has been introduced in Brazil since the First Republic (1889-1930), when Oswaldo Cruz was in charge of Brazil's public health administration. At that time, there were already interventions to control food risks, which were based on science and operationalized in the form of coercive measures (SOUTO, 2004).

Thus, the foundation of food health regulation, built from the ground up, remains practically intact, and is based on three pillars: regulation, inspection and control. In addition, it continues to encompass a set of legal instruments and technical-operational procedures that the competent public authority uses to govern the conduct of companies in the production, distribution and provision of services for different foodstuffs, with the aim of protecting the health of the population.

The current legal framework applied to food health control includes legal instruments from the last five decades. The oldest legal instrument, still in force, used as a reference in food health surveillance is Decree-Law No.º 986, of October 21, 1969, which establishes general rules on food and delegates responsibility for control to the Ministry of Health and similar state bodies. Approved by the military ministers of the Armed Forces, in a context of political dictatorship, the instrument brings together a set of control and inspection measures (registration, control analysis, licensing for establishments, among others), with the aim of checking that food products comply with the rules, and establishing penalties in the event of non-compliance with these rules.

At the time of its publication, extreme antagonistic events shared the same social scenario. On the one hand, the euphoria of economic flourishing and, on the other, the repression of individual freedoms, the concentration of income and the impoverishment of a large part of the population. According to Prado Jr (1988), the expansion of Brazilian industrialization was focused especially on consumer goods for the middle and upper classes and on raw materials and foodstuffs demanded by international markets. Encouraged by foreign capital, industrialization generated revenues that paid for the imports essential to our subsistence and the services provided by the imperialist oligopolies, which supported industrialization and national economic development. In the period 1968-71, the rate of growth of the food industry was 7.5% per year, but almost half of the volume produced (45.3%) (SUZIGAN et al, 1974 apud SINGER, 1976) met external demand (SINGER, 1976).

However, in order to facilitate foreign acceptance of food items, it was necessary to demonstrate to the foreign market the effectiveness of the country's sanitary control, with official rules established for food production, with definitions of identity and quality standards[22] of the products, containing hygiene parameters, among other aspects.

In reality, Decree-Law 986/69 was nothing new. It was simply a matter of improving some of the provisions of the previous rule and providing the sanitary control services with bureaucratic rationality, in order to speed up the demands of the expanding industrial sector (COSTA, 1999). As a result, the technical and legal apparatus was intensified, reorganizing sanitary control practices aimed at the food production sector, under the guidance of legislation based on product registration, inspection and the exercise of police power.

The country's interest in consolidating its position in the international food market was duly expressed at two points in the body of this Decree: a) in the provision authorizing the use of the international normative order in situations where there are no local norms and standards for the identity and quality of specific food products and; b) when it authorizes the manufacture of products for export in the country that comply exclusively with the rules of the country of destination. In short, this legislation represents an improvement in sanitary control and was one of the preparatory steps for the country's inclusion as a member of the FAO/WHO *Codex Alimentarius Commission*, so that it could participate in international food standardization, a fact that occurred as early as the 1970s (BRASIL; INMETRO, 2000).

With the political opening and the fundamental work of the social movements in the 1980s, especially the strategic Health Reform movement, which brought together progressive and popular sectors, the fight for *the right to health as a state guarantee, for decent living conditions (food, housing, income, employment, leisure, work, etc.) and for universal access to health promotion, protection and recovery services* were raised.[a]*) and for universal and equal access to health promotion, protection and recovery actions and*

22 Item XI of Article 10 of Chapter I of Decree-Law 986/69 establishes the following definition of "standard of identity and quality: that established by the competent body of the Ministry of Health, laying down the name, definition and composition of foods, food raw materials, foods *in natura* and intentional additives, establishing hygiene requirements, packaging and labeling standards measured by sampling and analysis".

services [...], enshrined in the 8th National Health Conference (BRASIL; MS, 1986, p.4).).

Between political struggles and clashes, the process of democratization of Brazilian society took shape, until the democratic rule of law was established with the advent of the 1988 Federal Constitution. The health reform movement played a strategic role in the approval of the Health chapter of the current Constitution, managing to materialize relevant social conquests, after overcoming certain resistance and pressure (ROSAS, 1988). During the constituent process, health surveillance was highlighted and definitively removed from its secondary status in the field of health, being mentioned in the proposed contribution to the constitutional text. As a result, the Constitution established that the Unified Health System is responsible for *carrying out health surveillance activities (...)* and for *inspecting and monitoring food, including the control of its nutritional content, as well as beverages and water for human consumption* (BRASIL; CONASS, 2003a, art. 200, items II and VI, CF).

Comparing the constitutional text with the current Decree-Law 986/69, there are two major innovations that enhance and expand the practice of health surveillance. The first is not to reduce this health practice to the mere exercise of police power, but to introduce, side by side, the action of **inspecting** and the action of **monitoring**. **Inspection** has an eminently technical meaning and is designed to assess the physical and functional conditions of the company in order to identify risk situations that could compromise the quality of the end product and cause harm to the health of the individual. The enforcement action is to force compliance with the rules. These actions complement each other and qualify the practice of health surveillance in technical, legal and effective terms. The second was the inclusion of the obligation to carry out *nutritional control.* This competence has not yet been properly explored in the field of health surveillance, but now, in view of the implication of food products in NCDs, it is opportune to evaluate the nutritional content of food products, in terms of calories and nutrient profile.

The Organic Health Law, Law No.º 8080, of September 19, 1990, subsequently approved, improved the advances contained in the text of the Constitution, and instituted the Unified Health System, which gave health surveillance the following definition:

a set of actions capable of eliminating, reducing or preventing health risks and intervening in health problems arising from the environment, the production and circulation of goods and the provision of services of interest to health, covering: the control of consumer goods that are directly or indirectly related to health, including all stages and processes, from production to consumption; and the control of the provision of services that are directly or indirectly related to health.

According to Costa (2013), the Constitution incorporated an expanded concept of health and the Organic Health Law was responsible for demarcating the space of health surveillance within the production-consumption relationship, giving it essentially preventive functions and reducing the risks of diseases and illnesses, and increasing its relevance in the field of health. As a result, the author clarifies that the field of action of health regulation and surveillance has grown in complexity and scope, both in terms of the type of risks and the conflicts of interest surrounding regulatory activities.

From that moment on, the primary objective of health surveillance is the prevention and control of health risks of any kind arising from economic activities of interest to health. To this end, it is up to public agents to combine technical and legal knowledge in order to deal with the dynamism of the risks that emerge from different sources and thus make it possible to defend the health of the public. Intervening in risks means, first and foremost, anticipating failures in the production process, applying measures to avoid damage or even to prevent it from spreading.

Another important step was the transfer of health surveillance activities to Anvisa at the end of the 90s. Law No.⁰ 9782, of January 26, 1999, delegates to this authority the responsibility for regulating, controlling and inspecting products and services that involve risks to public health, including foodstuffs and inputs, additives, packaging and contaminants and residues, as well as the physical and functional facilities responsible for processing such products - a subject that will be addressed in a later section.

In the light of the above, the process of normative construction of food health surveillance, which extends from Decree-Law No.⁰ 986/69 to the Organic Health Law, has seen substantial changes in its conception and practice: a) regulating goes beyond the simple act of regulating and inspecting, insofar as establishing rules and verifying compliance are insufficient to control risks; b) controlling the risk to health is the key; To this end, the introduction of a set of other technical-scientific actions in the practice of health surveillance is essential, which does not imply the abandonment or belittling of police power, but rather its strengthening by combining science with legal bases and; c) covering all health risks without distinction as to their nature, whether they are physical, chemical or biological contaminants, as well as those that are now emerging, the nutritional components of food.

In short, between the "anachronistic" and the "modern", or the "authoritarian" and the "democratic", the legal instruments come together to form the framework of food health regulation in Brazil. It is through day-to-day practice that the fusion of these two modalities comes to fruition and, in this way, the failures or tricks employed by the market are evaluated, circumvented and repressed, and the aim is to achieve what has been prescribed by law since the 1960s: the defense and protection of the health of the public against the risks arising from food production activity. This health action is the exclusive prerogative of the state and has been recognized and preserved throughout history, from militarism to democracy.

5.1.1 *Late 1990s: food regulation is the subject of the new authority*

Until 1998, the Ministry of Health distributed two technical functions among its administrative units to deal with food issues: one responsible for nutritional aspects and related health problems, and the other for the sanitary regulation of food and related products affecting public health. In the following year, the latter function was passed on to Anvisa, a federal authority which was given the task of regulating the market for all objects of interest to health.

The creation of the institutional figure of an autarchy under a special regime or regulatory agency was the result of the regulatory policies developed in Brazil during this decade, which were being molded to the American and European institutional standards implemented in the 1970s and 1980s respectively (RIBEIRO; COSTA; SILVA, 2000). In addition, the country received a lot of encouragement from international cooperation and funding bodies, which supported privatization and a change in the model of state intervention, as one of the ways to lead to national development (CRUZ, 2009). These organizations defined a system of disciplinary instructions that the government had to follow in order to obtain loans, support and technical assistance.

Adherence to the international agenda, combined with the fiscal crisis and limited resources for domestic investment, prompted the reform of the state, which dealt differently with economic and administrative aspects. On the economic front, it focused on the privatization of public companies and service providers and on formal and bureaucratic deregulation, with the aim of increasing competitiveness and economic efficiency. In the administrative sphere, especially in terms of institutional organization, it opted to reformulate the organizational model, creating specialized institutions, expanding their management capacity, developing regulatory structures and increasing the degree of accountability (GOMES, 2006; RIBEIRO; COSTA & SILVA, 2000). In short, the intention was to help build the most competitive market possible and to introduce business logic into the public sphere.

Bresser Pereira (1999, p.6-7), the intellectual mentor and driver of the managerial reform, argues that this new model of organization [...] *makes bureaucratic processes and regulations more flexible, giving a higher degree of autonomy and accountability to government agencies and their managers*, one of the means of which is the

[...] *management by objectives, the creation of quasi-markets and the various mechanisms of direct democracy or social control, combined with increased transparency in the public service, while at the same time reducing the role of the detailed definition of procedures and of auditing or internal control - the classic controls of bureaucratic public administration - which should be given less weight.*

In this sense, the agencies have taken over the activities that fall into the category of being exclusive to the state, which cannot be delegated, and which concern regulation, security and tax collection. Known as Regulatory Agencies, these autonomous, self-governing entities have a profile marked by administrative and financial autonomy, an emphasis on technical specialization and bureaucratic isolation[23] of their directors - who have fixed terms of office and stability in the exercise of their functions after a short term, among other requirements. This is in an attempt to keep the board distanced from the influences of the economic agents and political actors circulating in the sector.

These agencies then start to take care of regulation, which in itself encompasses a diverse set of instruments that the government uses to define the rules of conduct for companies and citizens in the economic, administrative and social fields. They aim to identify market failures at an early stage in the collective interest, such as negative externalities and a lack of information for consumers about the quality of the products and services offered by the market. However, it is social regulation[24] that is the focus of this study. This is because it is one of the spheres that refers to public intervention in the field of health, both to guarantee the provision of public goods and to protect the national or supranational

23 In this case, the term of office is three years, with a single reappointment. Unmotivated dismissal takes place only in the first four months of the mandate, except in cases of administrative misconduct, final criminal conviction and unjustified non-compliance with the agency's management contract. Former directors are prohibited from representing any person or interest before the Agency until one year after leaving office (RIBEIRO, COSTA & SILVA, 2000).

24 Social regulation is one of the three categories of regulation proposed by the Organization for Economic Cooperation and Development (OECD), which covers three specific fields: health, the environment and administration (CRUZ 2009).

public interest (COSTA et al, 2001), as it aims to reduce the harmful effects generated by the economic agents responsible for the production of goods of interest to health.

Although the official discourse addressed to public opinion emphasized that the ultimate aim of rebuilding the state was to make it capable of enabling economic development, protecting social and republican rights and strengthening democracy (BRESSER-PEREIRA, 1999), Cruz (2009) states that, in the case of the administrative reform, the most important arguments were the delegation of powers to the Regulatory Agencies, as well as the need to increase the degree of commitment by the public authorities to maintaining decisions and rules that directly affect agents. Thus, the private sector's positive attitude towards this type of reform is not surprising, since the initiatives seek to produce a reassuring institutional climate, with stability in the rules, an increase in the resolving capacity brought about by administrative autonomy and a reduction in the bureaucracy of internal processes, which helps to speed up the requests made by this sector.

It is worth noting that, at the time of the reform, the wear and tear on the institutional image of the federal health surveillance agency also served as a justification. After the political opening, the press exposed successive scandals involving food and medicines, disputes over economic and political interests and other administrative irregularities which, together with internal weaknesses in terms of qualified staff, inefficiency at work, limited resources, reduced autonomy, discredit in the ministerial sphere, among other aspects (SOUTO, 2004), made up the picture of the chaos in this sector.

As a counterpoint, there were also the demands of social movements and the new legal framework of the Organic Health Law, which forced institutional responses from health surveillance that were compatible with the interests of citizens, who wanted their health to be protected against inappropriate market practices. Thus, the sector's failure to act in accordance with its strategic role in health prevention, mainly due to its slowness in responding to market demands, strengthened the arguments of those in favor of administrative reform and its rapid extension to this sector (SOUTO, 2004).

Among the list of autarchies set up under a special regime, Anvisa was the fourth, approved by Federal Law No.º 9782 of January 26, 1999. The management reform led to a split between policy formulation and implementation. The former remained centralized in the strategic core of the government, while the latter was decentralized to the agencies (BRESSER PEREIRA, 2008). Anvisa, as part of the indirect administration of the health sector, is now linked to the Ministry of Health. However, it is an agency without hierarchical subordination, endowed with technical expertise and political credibility, to assume the role of regulating the production, marketing and distribution of products and services of interest to health, including food, as well as supervising - correcting, limiting or suspending - activities that threaten the health of the community; however, its primary function is to manage risks (CARVALHEIRO, 2001).

In order to strengthen the sectoral ministries vis-à-vis the agencies, an additional instrument for social control and for improving the management and performance of the regulatory agencies was created - the management contract (GOMES, 2006). In this case, this contract is the result of a negotiation of health interests between Anvisa's collegiate board and the Minister of Health, whose execution reports and annual rendering of accounts are presented to the competent bodies and the National Health Council (BRASIL; ANVISA, 2006a).

Another special feature of Anvisa is its role in coordinating the group of similar bodies in the states and municipalities that make up the National Health Surveillance System (SNVS). This system is interconnected to the Unified Health System (SUS) and follows the principles of decentralization and integration. Its members carry out similar tasks, with a direct impact on the population, except for those that fall under the restricted competence of Anvisa, such as granting registration of food products with national validity. With relative autonomy and independence, the state entities can move forward with proposals for food control and risk management that respond more effectively to the demands of the local reality, without being subject solely to the deliberations of the federal entity.

Considering the neoliberal precepts that underpinned the creation of the agencies, one of the central issues raised when Anvisa was created was its tendency to favor the demands of the business community (reducing bureaucracy, regulations, etc.), to the detriment of the collective need to control the risks of products, especially when these imply confrontations with the former. Various experiences in the field of food show that ANVISA's conduct has not been at odds with private interests, but has neglected the interests of society. Examples include: (*i*) waiving the obligation to register food products, without compensating for this with a concrete reinforcement of inspection activities in industries and food control, to keep them under surveillance; (*ii*) abolishing the rules that establish the identity parameters of food products, leaving the consumer without a reference for the composition of the product; (*iii*) failure to set up an information system accessible to the entire health surveillance network, allowing simultaneous exchange of information and rapid action by the health authorities in the face of product/service risks; (*iv*) failure to control food advertising to children.

However, the reform of public management set out to be innovative in terms of the practice of governance. Governed by the key actor government, this practice is used to support government decisions and allow it to act together with other social actors, making the process of governing participatory and democratic (BRESSER PEREIRA, 2008). It is therefore appropriate for organized civil society to be included within the institutes, in order to give plurality of voices in the public spaces that debate and define the direction of decisions.

A few years after its creation, the government assessed the need for improvement, seeking to adjust the functioning of the agencies in terms of the development of instruments for social control and the role of these institutions in the Brazilian administrative structure (BRASIL; CASA CIVIL, 2003). To this end, Anvisa has introduced into its structures information procedures, public hearings and public consultations, channels for a participatory management process, a space for sharing collective discussions between the interested parties - citizens, industrialists and the government - in order to seek consensus between the various interests, whether through alliances and partnerships or the management of conflicts and disputes of interest. In Lucchese's (2001) opinion, a space has been created for the exercise of citizenship and social control which, aided by the interdisciplinary and inter-institutional action of health surveillance and the adoption of ethical parameters to guide the production-consumption relationship, can be used to transform the quality of products, processes and social relations in order to satisfy collective interests.

In order to improve regulatory practices, Anvisa's organizational structure also included a body for the institutionalized participation of society, called the Consultative Council[25] (BRASIL; ANVISA, 2005). In 2009, a mechanism was introduced to rationalize and simplify the regulatory process, as well as consolidate and revise normative acts, which is the Regulatory Agenda (RA) (BRASIL; ANVISA, 2012). As a pioneering initiative by the federal public administration, this agenda has a four-year cycle and two two-year

---

25 The Advisory Council is one of Anvisa's instruments for social participation, made up of representatives of the Union, States, Municipalities, the Federal District, producers, traders, the scientific community and organized civil society, with the aim of giving opinions on the institution's government policy proposals, requesting information and proposing recommendations and technical guidelines on matters relating to the Agency, among other issues (BRASIL; ANVISA, 2005).

agendas, made up of issues considered strategic and priority and previously discussed with representatives of civil society, the regulated sector and the National Health Surveillance System in order to achieve *[...] benefits such as predictability, transparency, governance, a commitment to greater efficiency and credibility for the regulatory process* (BRASIL; ANVISA, 2010, p.36).

The first two-year period (2013-1014) of the Quadrennial Cycle (2013-2016)[26] of the RA included 23 themes related to the area of food and, among the list, theme[0] 19, which refers to the *Advertising of Foods with High Quantities of Sugar, Saturated Fat, Trans Fat, Sodium and Beverages with Low Nutritional Content,* is the one that has an interface with the subject of this thesis and will be revisited below. This issue has resurfaced for debate, with the support of organized civil society, due to the obesity epidemic and the increase in the prevalence of other CNCDs that are already affecting the child population. In the past, rules have been approved but failed to be implemented due to legal obstacles. The action of civil society will therefore be decisive in achieving the expected success - which is to discipline, or even restrict, the dissemination of this type of advertising to children.

Certainly, agencies have structures with greater flexibility and capacity to adapt to the dynamism of the globalized world, due to their normative and executive potential, and their openness to the participation of organized civil society in the exercise of their mission (PECI, 1999). As far as Anvisa is concerned, the technical specialization and spaces for society's participation that are being built, with the maturity experienced by the entity, can project advances in the process of democratization of decisions on how to intervene in the health risks of objects under the control of health surveillance. However, the journey is still long, requires caution and is subject to setbacks. The improvement of Anvisa's activities depends fundamentally on the active and qualified participation of organized civil society, as well as its commitment and external coordination, in order to become a social force on a par with the market and public power. In this way, the Regulatory Agenda can change and start to focus on issues that are relevant to the community in terms of protecting and controlling health risks.

---

26 The drafting of the RA begins with a prior consultation of various strategic government documents: the 2012-15 Multiannual Plan, the report of the 14th National Health Conference, the Brasil Sem Miséria and Brasil Maior guidelines and plans, the National Health Plan and the Health Surveillance Master Plan (PDVISA), institutional strategic planning and guidelines from the Board of Directors, among other documents. The RA has a Quadrennial Cycle (2013-2016) and two regulatory agendas, each valid for two years. The one for the 2013-2014 biennium contains priority issues for Anvisa's regulatory activities: 148 themes divided into 14 macro-themes. This RA, published in the DOU on September 24, 2013, represents the first publication of the new model (BRASIL; ANVISA, 2012).

5.2 Anvisa and the Ministry of Health: institutional (re)action

As a result of the current epidemiological picture of nutritional deficiencies, obesity and CNCDs, concern about the quality of food at national level has become the object of attention in two sectors of the federal public administration; the General Coordination of Food and Nutrition of the Department of Basic Care of the Secretariat of Health Care of the Ministry of Health - CGAN/DAB/MS and the General Food Management of the National Health Surveillance Agency - GGALI/Anvisa/MS. The former is responsible for implementing the National Food and Nutrition Policy (PNAN), and Anvisa's agenda is related to the sanitary control of foodstuffs under this policy.

The PNAN-1999 represents the first sectoral nutrition policy and was based on the results of the First National Conference on Food Security in 1994. Its content already mentioned the broadening of nutritional problems with the inclusion of the evolution of the obesity epidemic, dyslipidemia and its relationship with cardiovascular diseases, as well as those of a deficiency nature. It emphasized the responsibility of the state to promote and facilitate the means for individuals to have a decent diet, contributing to a healthy and active life and to the realization of the Human Right to Adequate Food (BRASIL; MS, 1999).

In the updated version of the 2012 PNAN (BRASIL; MS, 2012a), two guidelines stand out for guiding the practice of food quality control: "Food control and regulation" and "Promoting adequate and healthy food". For the first guideline, food regulation actions should focus on the safety and nutritional quality of food. The second guideline, linked to the first, focuses on the importance of food meeting biological needs at each stage of the life cycle, according to gender, race and ethnicity, while also observing other principles such as respect for food culture; physical and financial accessibility; adequate and sustainable production practices; quantitative and qualitative harmony, among other aspects, with a view to improving quality of life and reducing excess weight and diseases related to food and nutrition.

The pioneering experiences of the newly created Anvisa with the Ministry of Health to meet the provisions of the PNAN were firstly related to the directive *Prevention and control of nutritional disorders and diseases associated with food and nutrition and*, as part of the Program to Combat Iodine Deficiency Disorders in Brazil (BRASIL; ANVISA, 2000), new limits for iodine in salt were approved, good practice rules were established for salt processing establishments and a national health inspection program for these establishments was instituted (BRASIL; ANVISA, 2004). This was followed by the approval of limits for folic acid and iron in wheat and corn flours (BRASIL; ANVISA, 2002), with subsequent monitoring of these products. In 2001, considering the PNAN/1999 guideline *Guaranteeing the safety and quality of food and the provision of services in this context* - which proposes updating the rules and procedures of health surveillance, including nutritional labeling - the rules for mandatory nutritional labeling of packaged foods and beverages were published (BRASIL; ANVISA, 2001). These labelling rules were later republished as a result of the harmonization of their content within Mercosur.

In 2005, a multisectoral working group was set up at the National Health Surveillance Agency (Anvisa/MS) to deal with the 1999 PNAN guideline *Promoting healthy eating practices and lifestyles.* On that occasion, it was proposed to regulate the advertising of children's food products, above all in partnership with entities representing the advertising sector, organized civil society and the production sector and communications companies. This resulted in the publication of an Anvisa Public Consultation No. 71/2006, which deals with the supply, advertising and publicity of foods with high amounts of sugar, saturated fat, *trans* fat and sodium (BRASIL; ANVISA, 2006b). After four years of intense debate, ANVISA Resolution-RDC No. 24/2010 was approved, but with its content softened compared to the text of the Public Consultation (BRASIL; ANVISA, 2010b). However, the clashes in the Judiciary resulted in it losing its legal effectiveness, due to the controversy created by industries, communication and advertising companies.

Based on this list of joint activities between the Ministry of Health and Anvisa, a number of considerations can be made: a) the sanitary control of food is not dissociated from nutritional issues, considering Anvisa's precipitous function of protecting the population against the risks of food; and this has proven to be part of the institutional routine of the entity since its creation; b) the food products in question were adjusted to the nutritional requirements, by establishing rules with sanctions allied to systematic control measures to check their suitability and; c) the national industries involved were obliged to pay for the addition of nutrients (iron and folic acid or iodine) to the products considered essential to meet the official nutrition programs.

As the epidemiological panorama worsened, revealing the advance of CNCDs and the increase in health care costs and their association with the change in the dietary pattern of the Brazilian population, due to the increase in the availability of unhealthy foods, among other aspects, the government was ready to react. In 2007, the Ministry of Health, following international recommendations, set up a Technical Group under its coordination, with initial representation from the government and industry, to discuss and propose actions aimed at improving the supply of food products and promoting healthy eating (BRASIL; MS, 2007b). Following this, a cooperation agreement was signed between the Ministry of Health and the Brazilian Association of Food Industries (ABIA) and a public call was approved to assess the potential of the production sector to gradually reduce the levels of various nutrients in processed foods, such as free sugar, *trans* fats, saturated fats and salt (BRASIL; MS, 2007c), which culminated in several subsequent terms of commitment, as shown in Table 2.

TABLE 2: Instruments of cooperation signed between the Ministry of Health and entities representing the food industry between 2007 and 2014.

MS and Industry Cooperation Instrument/Date	Purpose / Obligations	Competence Highlights
1. Cooperation Agreement Technical meeting between MS and ABIA 29/11/2007	Joining forces to implement actions Joint efforts to promote lifestyles which includes a healthy, balanced and nutritionally adequate diet.	(MS)To set up, by means of a separate act, a Technical Group for the purpose of propose a gradual strategy for reducing free sugar content. sodium, saturated fats and *trans* fatty acids in processed foods; **(MS)** Establish a gradual strategy to improve the nutritional profile of industrialized foods, with the focus described above; **(ABIA)** To recommend, together with media organizations, ethical and responsible practices for the marketing and advertising of food and non-alcoholic drinks.
2. Term of extension of the agreement between the MS and ABIA 25/11/2010	Joining forces to implement actions joint efforts to promote healthy lifestyles, which includes healthy, balanced and nutritionally adequate food.	Extend for 3 (three) years, starting from the expiry date of the Technical Cooperation Agreement.
3 Term of Commitment No. 004/2011 between MS and ABIA, ABIMA, ABITRIGO and ABIP 07/04/2011	Establishing national targets for the reduction of sodium content in processed foods in the Brazil Institutions commit to reducing o	**(MS)** Implement the National Plan to Reduce Health Consumption, through voluntary reductions in processed foods and Food preparations in food and beverage establishments restaurants; increasing the supply of healthy food, labeling

Term: 3 years	maximum sodium level in food categories Industrialized: macaroni other Categories (French bread, ready-made cakes, cake mixes, corn snacks and French fries, sausages, broths and dressings, cereal derivatives, laticinios, ready-made meals and cookies), in order to subsequently set targets for sodium reduction.	and consumer information, etc. Coordinate the activities of the WG and monitor the evolution of sodium content in food categories. **(ABIA, ABIMA, ABITRIGO and ABIP)** Articulate with the food industries in each category to adhere to the pact; encourage the implementation of quality control systems and monitoring of sodium content in food; contribute to monitoring the sodium content of target foods and develop and commit to technologies for reducing sodium content.

TABLE 2: Cooperation instruments signed between the Ministry of Health and entities representing food industries between 2007 and 2014 (Continued**).**

MS and industry cooperation instrument/Date	Purpose / Obligations	Competence Highlights
4. Agreement of Cooperation Technique between o MSeaABRAS- 07/04/2011 Deadline duration: 3 years.	Meeting forces and working Jointly to implement actions Aimed at promoting the quality of life and prevention factors determinants and/or constraints of diseases and health problems.	**(MS)** Draw up strategies in cooperation with ABRAS aimed at promoting quality of life and the prevention of determining and/or conditioning factors of diseases and health problems, prioritizing aspects of nutrition healthy, body practices/physical activity, health control smoking, reducing the abuse of alcohol and other drugs, reducing the damage caused by traffic accidents and encouraging a culture of peace; strengthening institutional public health campaigns, in partnership with ABRAS; ABRAS may join other Working Groups formally set up by the Ministry of Health, especially those related to improving the nutritional profile of processed foods and its own manufacturing lines. **(ABRAS)** To promote, together with its members, education and information activities and campaigns to promote quality of life, as agreed in the Technical Group; to recommend to its members the adoption of internal policies for quality control of raw materials and selection of suppliers; recommend, together with media organizations,

		ethical practices for the responsible *marketing and* advertising of food and beverages; implement actions to promote health and quality of life for workers in food establishments.

TABLE 2: Instruments of cooperation signed between the Ministry of Health and the entities representing the food industries between 2007 and 2014. (Continued)

Instrument of MS and industry cooperation/Date	Purpose/Obligations	Competence Highlights
5. ***Term of Commitment between MS, ABIA,*** *ABIMA, ABITRIGO* ***andABip*** **13/12/2011.** ***Term: 5 years***	Setting national targets for the reduction of sodium content in processed foods in Brazil The institutions undertake to reduce the maximum level of sodium in the following categories food Industrialized products: French bread, ready-made cakes with or without filling, rocambole, aerated cake, creamy cake mixes, corn snacks, potato chips and straws, mayonnaise, sweet cookies, savory cookies and filled cookies.	**(MS)** Implement the National Plan for Reducing Sodium Consumption, through voluntary reductions in industrialized foods and preparations sold in food establishments and restaurants; increasing the supply of healthy foods, labelling and consumer information, etc. Coordinate the activities of the WG and monitor the evolution of sodium content in food categories. **(ABIA, ABIMA, ABITRIGO and ABI?)** Articulate with the food industries in each category to join the pact; encourage the implementation of quality control systems and monitoring of sodium content in food; contribute to monitoring the sodium content of target foods and develop and commit to technologies for reducing sodium content.
6. ***Term of Commitment between MS and ABIA*** **28/08/2012.** ***Term: 3 years***	Setting national targets for the reduction of sodium content in processed foods in Brazil The institutions undertake to reduce the maximum level of sodium in the following categories food Industrialized: cereal derivatives, vegetable margarine, liquid and gel broths, paste seasonings, rice seasonings and other seasonings.	**(MS)** Implement the National Plan for Reducing Sodium Consumption, through voluntary reductions in industrialized foods and food preparations in food establishments and restaurants; increasing the supply of healthy foods, labelling and consumer information, etc. Coordinate the activities of the WG and monitor the evolution of sodium content in food categories. **(ABIA, ABIMA, ABITRIGO and ABIP)** Articulate with the food industries in each category to adhere to the pact; encourage the implementation of quality control systems and monitoring of sodium content in food; contribute to monitoring the sodium content of target foods and develop and commit to technologies for reducing sodium content.

TABLE 2: Cooperation instruments signed between the Ministry of Health and

entities representing food industries between 2007 and 2014 (Continued).

MS and industries cooperation agreement/Date	Purpose/Obligations	Competence Highlights
7. *Term of commitment to ABIA, ABIC, ABIPECS, SINCARNES and UBABEF 0S/11/2013. Term: 3 years, extendable for an equal period.*	Agree on strategies for the food industry to contribute to reducing the consumption of sai by the Brazilian population to less than 5g of sai per person per day by 2020, by reducing the sodium content in priority categories (laticinios, soups and meat products available for consumption and processed foods).	**(MS)** Implement the National Sodium Consumption Reduction Plan, through the following axes: (i) voluntary reduction of sodium levels in processed foods and preparations sold in food establishments and restaurants; (ii) increasing the supply of healthy foods; (iii) labeling and consumer information and (iv) education and awareness-raising for consumers, industry, health professionals and other stakeholders. **(ABIA, ABIC, ABIPECS, SINDICARNES and UBABEF)** Articulate the industries in each category to commit to the process of agreeing targets for reducing sodium in processed foods; encourage the implementation of quality control systems and monitoring of sodium content in foods.
8. *Cooperation agreement between o MS and ABIA 24/01/2014. Term: 3 years, extendable for an equal period.*	0I n Pooling efforts and work Jointly to implement actions, in order to articulate the form of collaboration between the parties for the effective execution of the National Healthy Living Piano, covering aspects of food, healthy nutrition, physical activity and education; ensure the population's access to adequate food, Select Institutional campaigns among others.	To extend the term of the Technical Cooperation Agreement for 3 (three) years.

The Agreement was then a milestone for discussing the reduction of the nutritional parameters of products considered unhealthy, which began with the mobilization for the removal of *trans* fats from products, where important progress was only made in 2010 (BRASIL; MS, 2012b).

At the same time, the National Council for Food and Nutritional Security (CONSEA)[27] drew

27 CONSEA was created in April 1993 as an advisory body to the Presidency of the Republic on matters related to food and nutrition security.

up a proposal for an intersectoral strategy to promote adequate and healthy food. In this proposal, food is approached from a macro perspective, encompassing socio-economic, cultural and biological aspects, and is reaffirmed as a basic individual right to a healthy life, the viability of which depends on the valorization of food sovereignty and the recovery of traditional and sustainable production practices. The strategy included actions involving different institutional actors, such as promoting the consumption of legumes, fruit and vegetables, regulating the advertising of food products high in saturated fat, *trans* fat, sugar, sodium and drinks with low nutritional value (BRASIL; CONSEA, 2007).

In 2009, Anvisa/MS coordinated a diagnosis to assess the nutritional composition of 24 types of industrialized food, in terms of sodium, sugar, saturated fat, *trans* fat and iron content. The result revealed a discrepant variation in sodium content between foods in the same category. In the case of instant noodles and noodle seasoning, the highest amounts of sodium per portion were found, which in themselves already exceed the daily reference value of 2400mg/day. The sugar levels detected in soft drinks, juice and nectar were close to the average values of between 10 and 11.7g/100mL. This shows that if an individual drinks a regular glass (200mL) of soft drink, they are consuming an average of 20g of sugar. As for the saturated fat content, the highlights were French fries and straws with an average of 3.5 and 3.8 g/25g of portion and filled and salted cookies with an average of 1.6/30g of portion (BRASIL; ANVISA, 2010). Comparing the average sugar and fat levels found in these foods with the classification and weight/volume criteria established by the UK's food standards agency[28] , all these products had high levels, and could fall into the "high sugar" or "high fat" categories.

These results are worrying because the food products highlighted are commonly consumed by children who, in addition to the negative health effects of high sodium, sugar and fat consumption, encourage the formation of consumption habits that adapt the palate to prefer foods with this nutritional composition. As a result of this diagnosis, the health authorities made subsequent negotiations with industry organizations to first reduce the sodium content in various categories of food (Table 2), despite the fact that the

28 The United Kingdom's Food Standards Agency is recommending that the front of the packaging of certain processed products be affixed with a nutritional signpost, indicating the sugar, fat, saturated fat and salt content in different colors. The products were selected on the basis of a survey of consumers who said they found it difficult to evaluate certain categories of products in nutritional terms. Thus, the limits that categorize products as high in sugar for liquid products and high in fat for solid products are respectively greater than 6.3g/100mL and greater than 5g/100g (UNITED KINDOWN, 2007).

epidemiological picture indicates an urgent need to reduce all nutrients. The reference value for defining the reduction target, in the absence of an equivalent international reference, was based on three sources: the lower limit of the sodium content indicated by the results of the diagnosis, in those types of food then analyzed; the information on the label; and the information provided by the industries. The Ministry of Health's aim is to reduce sodium consumption by the Brazilian population to less than 2000mg/person/day by 2020 (BRASIL; MS, 2011).

In 2011, the Ministry of Health launched the "Strategic Action Plan for Tackling Chronic Non-Communicable Diseases (CNCD) in Brazil - 20112022", which brings together a set of effective and integrated public policies, under its leadership and with an intersectoral nature, to intervene in these diseases. Unhealthy diets are one of the risk factors that are being targeted. To this end, among other actions, it proposes agreements with industries to reduce salt and sugar in processed foods, increase the supply and reduce the prices of healthy foods and establish regulations on advertising to children (BRASIL; MS, 2011).

Meanwhile, motivated by the results confirming the uncontrolled increase in the prevalence of excess weight (POF 2008/09), a Technical Committee was set up within the Interministerial Chamber for Food and Nutritional Security - CAISAN/MDS, which formulated the Intersectoral Plan for the Prevention and Control of Obesity. It consists of six lines of action - one of which refers to "*Regulation and control of food quality and safety*", with the aim of improving nutritional quality, covering food advertising, nutritional labeling and adapting the nutritional profile of processed foods to what is considered healthy, among other aspects (BRASIL; MDS, 2012a). It was submitted to CONSEA in October 2012, but has not yet been officially launched. In the absence of official information on its development, the Intersectoral Strategy for the Prevention and Control of Obesity was released. In this document, part of the content presented in the Plan is approached from the perspective of the responsibilities of states and municipalities in the prevention and control of obesity.

In the National Congress, this issue is mainly dealt with by the Social Security and Family Committee of the Chamber of Deputies[29] , which is in charge of dealing with the matter that interfaces "food and health". In the period from 2000 to 2013, 41 bills - PL (Table 3)

---

29 According to the Internal Rules of the Chamber of Deputies, in article 32, item XII, one of this Commission's attributions is to deal with matters relating to health, welfare and social assistance in general; drug, medicine and food control; blood and blood products; drug, medicine and food control; blood and blood products; food and nutrition, among others (BRASIL; CÂMARA DOS DEPUTADOS, 2013).

- were processed on topics directly or indirectly linked to the content of this thesis. Most of them came from this Commission. But in the last year, three of them were presented by other committees: two, by the Consumer Protection Committee, item 12 (only the one referring to posters - PL 5469/13) and item 17 (PL 6985/13); and another, by the Agriculture, Livestock, Supply and Rural Development Committee (item 20). This is PL 58666/13, which proposes removing the following warning phrase from the label of infant formulas: *"This product should not be used to feed children under one (1) year of age. Breastfeeding prevents infections and allergies and is recommended until 2 (two) years of age or older"*, which aims to alert mothers/guardians to the benefits of breastfeeding over artificial milk. This bill, if approved, will represent a step backwards in the fight to encourage breastfeeding and healthy eating.

In summary, it is possible to group the subjects of the PLs into three large groups, according to their purpose: a) intervening in obesity - food education, campaigns and raising public awareness, publicizing the risks (items 1, 2, 5, 7, 10 and 12); b) intervening in products - restricting food advertising and publicity, providing information on nutrient and/or calorie content, reducing sugar, including health risk warnings on labeling, information on the caloric value of manipulated products by means of posters, nutritional labeling, prohibition of associating food products with gifts and the like (items 3, 4, 6, 9, 11, 12, 13, 14, 15, 17, 18) and; c) intervening in school food (8, 16 and 19). On the basis of these grouped matters, rules on school food, nutritional labeling and food education were produced, either within the Chamber of Deputies itself or on the initiative of the competent federal body. The only issue that didn't produce results was the one on food products, because the issue of food regulation directly clashes with the economic interests of the market - which are duly represented and strengthened in the "People's House".

TABLE 3: Bills presented in the Chamber of Deputies of the National Congress on topics of interest from 2000 to 2013.

Nº	Material	Quantity
1	Principles and guidelines for nutritional education actions and nutritional and food security for the population / Promotion of healthy eating. (PL: 1234/07; 3310/04; 6803/10)	3
2	Policy to combat obesity/ Obliges comprehensive care for patients in the SUS (PL: 1394/01; 1560/03; 1684/03; 1699/03; 6183/13)	5
3	Disclosure of obesity warnings on food products (PL: 1480/03)	1
4	Obliges commercial food establishments to display posters informing about the calories in each portion served. / Nutritional information on food for	2

	immediate consumption. (PL: 1790/03; 2714/03)	
5	Creates a week or day of national mobilization against obesity or to raise awareness about the harmful effects of obesity. (PL: 6086/02; 4438/04; 1965/11; 3652/12; 3874/12)	**5**
6	Restricting the advertising of drinks and foods that potentially cause obesity (PL: 6080/05; 1637/07; 3793/08; 4462/08; 7644/10; 5608/13)	**6**
7	Creates a program to prevent and guide the treatment of childhood obesity (PL: 6522/09)	**1**
8	Prohibits the sale and consumption of sweets in schools (PL: 6848/02)	**1**
9	Prohibits the use of highlighting quality and nutritional characteristics statements on food packaging and in food advertising. (PL: 5629/13)	**1**

TABLE 3: Bills presented in the Chamber of Deputies of the National Congress on topics of interest from 2000 to 2013 (Continued)

Nº	**Material**	**Quantity**
10	Inclusion of food education in primary and secondary school curricula (PL: 325/07)	**1**
11	Obliges warnings about disease risks on product labels and in commercial advertisements for foods high in sugar, saturated fat, *trans* fat, sodium and drinks with low nutritional content. (PL: 4705/01; 7667/10; 4803/12)	**3**
12	Obliges the use of obesity warning posters in establishments that sell "fast food." (PL: 5469/13; 5674/13) Obliges specifying the number of calories in food sold on menus in restaurants, cafeterias and the like.	**2**
13	Sets a maximum limit on the amount of sucrose added to commercialized juices / Reduces the sugar content of foods intended for children (PL: 5883/13; 6836/13)	**2**
14	It is abusive to offer gifts, toys, etc. associated with the purchase of food and drink for children. (PL: 6111/13)	**1**
15	Nutritional labeling of processed foods (PL: 3909/00)	**1**
16	Mandates healthy food in public and private elementary schools (PL: 3170/00)	**1**
17	Obliges commercialized food products to inform about the presence or absence of salt as a preventive measure against diseases. (PL: 6985/13)	**1**

TABLE 3: Bills presented in the Chamber of Deputies of the National Congress on topics of interest from 2000 to 2013 (Continued)

Nº	**Material**	**Quantity**
18	Regulates commercial advertising of products, practices and services aimed at children and adolescents. (PL: 6777/13)	**1**
19	Prohibits the sale of soft drinks to children under 18 and foods with high caloric value and low levels of nutrients in schools. (PL: 5043/13; 6283/13)	**2**

20	Repeals the compulsory warning on the labels of infant formula for children under the age of Iª (PL: 5866/13)	1
	TOTAL	**41**

Thus, the Legislative Branch, like the Executive Branch, had no interest in regulating the issue. The Ministry of Health then introduced a new instrument in the field of food control, which was the implementation of Agreements and their Terms of Commitment (items 2, 3, 5 and 7 in Table 2) signed between the government and the entities representing the industries, for the reduction of sodium. There are some drawbacks to this instrument: (*i*) great elasticity - the deadlines for reducing noise, for example, vary between 3 and 5 years; (*ii*) limited extension - the formality of the Agreement and the Terms are restricted to the entities representing the industries that have ratified them; and (*iii*) fragility in compliance - the lack of punitive clauses can delay compliance with these acts.

Thus, in order to infer the basis for the negotiation of the targets referred to in these Terms (items 3 and 5 of Table 2), the behavior of six food products in terms of the nutrient sodium obtained in the diagnosis was compared with the agreed reduction targets (Graph 1) and it was found that the targets for three products were defined by the highest value identified and for the other three, those closest to the highest value. The choice of flexibility in the targets shows that the government was quite lenient with the market when implementing these acts. This is possible because data shows that there is technical and commercial viability to speed up the reduction of sodium content in food products. Because, among the products monitored, there are some that are circulating on the market, whose formulas contain sodium content below the agreed reduction limit - hence it can be inferred that there is consumer acceptance and feasible technology for their production. This becomes more evident when the government, by choosing not to impose compulsory rules, "wastes" the opportunity to use the minimum sodium value found in the monitored products as a reference for building the basis of the Terms.

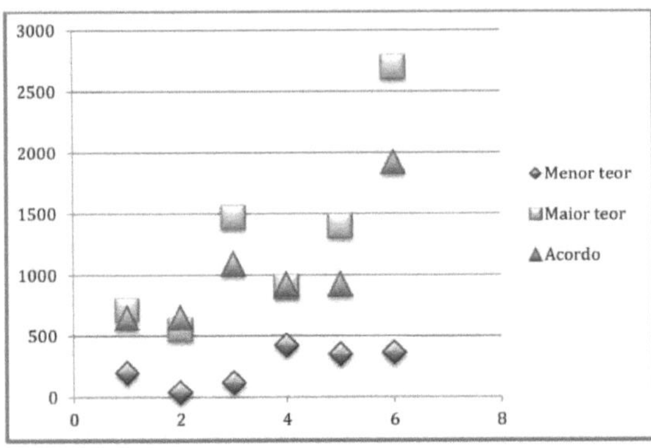

1 French fries

2 Straw potatoes

3 Corn snacks

4 Water and salt cookies

5 Cream cracker

6 Instant noodles.

Graph 1: Comparison between the sodium levels diagnosed in food products and the reduction values agreed between the government and the entities representing the food industry. Brazil, 2010-2011.

SOURCE: BRAZIL; ANVISA. Technical Report n. 42/2010; items 3 and 5 of Table 2.

Although compliance with Agreements and Terms of Commitment is being assumed in the institutional practice of health surveillance, discarding the use of regulation with negotiated and fixed deadlines and with provision for sanctions means weakening control measures and the role of authority and intervention by the state in private activity, aimed at making public interests prevail. In addition, the regulation is preceded by procedures of democratic construction, established within the competent regulatory agency, while the practice of the agreement is centralized and restricted. It should be noted that compliance with the agreement depends only on the degree of commitment between the parties, which does not in itself extend to other entities and companies in the sector. It is necessary for the public authorities to view the management of food risks related to obesity and other NCDs as equivalent to that applied to STDs, using the traditional resources (regulation, product monitoring, inspection of establishments, etc.), in order to achieve effective control of the nutritional quality of the food products involved.

However, it is worth pointing out that the fundamental difference in the effect of food risk management aimed at preventing CNCDs lies in the economic impacts claimed by the production sector, which have prompted a strong reaction from the market. This is because risk management implies reformulating the current concept of industrialized food production (low cost, high consumption and poor nutritional quality, designed with a focus on profits and without health benefits). It's important to note that the reactions of the food corporations have already made the Danish government back down, revoking the measures to tax products with a high saturated fat content (PETKANTCHIN, 2013), but, on the other hand, they weren't enough to stop the mobilized Finnish society from moving forward and forcing the reformulation of products, guaranteeing food with improved nutritional quality (PUSKA, 2004).

From the point of view of the Ministry of Health and Anvisa, there is an appreciation of this experience of government agreements with industry entities for the reduction of health, as being innovative, legitimate and transparent, based on intra-institutional articulation and with the private sector, and on the establishment of a dialogic and agreed relationship that strengthens social control (NILSON; JAIME; RESENDE, 2012). Without praising the vanguardism of institutional practice or dismissing the possible merits of this initiative, a few points need to be made: firstly, the ideological value of this measure, demonstrated by the government's concern for public health, is what stands out, given that it dispenses with the state's prerogatives to impose rules on the market and opts to make flexible, long-term agreements. Secondly, in order to strengthen social control, it is necessary for all of society's representatives to be involved in the discussions held in the public sphere and, in this case, the treatment given to civil society, the biggest stakeholder in the issue, was the complete exclusion from this negotiation process, even compromising the legitimacy referred to by the authors.

5.2.1 Partnership between government and industry: weakness or innovation

The Public-Private Partnership in the field of health[30] - PppS is a relatively new phenomenon and still lacks a precise definition. It may refer to some kind of engagement or interaction between the public and private sectors, or even to a relationship between them, established on the basis of strict criteria. This type of partnership is based on the sharing of objectives and, to some degree, decision-making between the public and private sectors. However, in general, there is no provision for the participation of non-profit organizations (HAWKES, 2008b).

30 In public health, this type of partnership is completely different from private contracts for the execution of public services signed in the form of Public-Private Partnerships (HAWKES, 2008b). In these cases, the government signs concession contracts with private partners, who are responsible for making investments in infrastructure and providing services of public interest, for a fixed term.

According to this author, the PPPs related to diet, nutrition and physical activity are being implemented more slowly than those involving medicines. The initiatives being adopted in various countries basically focus on four areas: improving food products (salt reduction), educating the public, nutrition labeling and advertising and, finally, research.

The formalization of the PppS, established on the basis of this joint work, seeks to achieve effective results, with a reduction in resources and political-institutional wear and tear, and is, in certain circumstances, more advantageous than a measure undertaken by the government alone. However, for partnerships to materialize into agreements, there is a process of negotiation to establish mutual responsibilities and shared interests, and it is essential to generate benefits for both parties, clearly explained in advance, in an environment of transparency and accountability, so that this alliance can be consolidated (MITCHELL, 2008). Thus, in the field of health, the governance of PHPP focuses on five key issues: representation, participation, accountability, transparency and effectiveness (HAWKES, 2008b).

From the 1990s onwards, the FAO and the WHO began to encourage countries to develop joint actions to deal with obesity and other CNCDs, by linking governments, industries and consumers (WHO, 1990). These organizations state that it is essential to create multisectoral strategies with different actors, on a long-term basis; to form alliances and partnerships; and to engage them in collaborative programs, since the responsibility for preventing these diseases is shared. However, the industry's responsibility is to improve the quality of its food products (WHO, 2000; WHO, 2002b; WHO, 2003b). They believe that the articulated action of public policy makers, producers, consumers and other partners can transform the character of the food system, making it "more compatible with nutritional precepts" (FAO, 2013b).

In Europe, numerous partnerships have been set up to tackle the phenomenon of overweight and obesity in the region, with the backing of the Commission of the European Communities, whose main target is consumers. Thus, very often, these partnerships are aimed at changing consumer behavior, providing them with information to review their consumption habits and physical exercise habits, viewing obesity as an individual problem within a conservative-liberal conception rather than instigating structural changes that determine these behaviors (BORCH; ROOS, 2012). There are also partnerships aimed at reducing the unhealthy components of food (HAWKES, 2008b).

The challenge is to harmonize interests, within the "naturally" installed divergences between the agents of the production sector, which aims for private profit and the trade in food products (hypercaloric and high in sodium), and public agents, invested with the precipitous function of protecting the interests of the community. In the case of Brazil, despite the existence of these differences, it is possible that the systematic warnings issued by international organizations, the government and local media about the risks of unhealthy food products, as well as a remote insecurity on the part of manufacturers about the use of a compulsory intervention measure - regulation -, have sensitized the corporate entities of the industries to commit themselves to negotiating with the government and thus avoid any instability in the trade of such products.

In order to deal with this food issue, the Brazilian government decided to use instruments such as "Agreements and Terms of Commitment", and renounced the path of regulation. The first impression is that these instruments seem to symbolize an administrative innovation, but in fact they represent a step backwards when compared to the democratic process of regulation that has been instituted within the framework of public institutes, allowing for a broad debate and the participation of organized sectors and society in general. It also demonstrates the government's weakness in managing food risks with the agility required and with the authority and competence attributed to it. The political difficulties are real, the reaction of the powerful market corporations is effective, but the vacuum imposed on civil society is indicative of contradictory conduct and a clear unwillingness to enlist the support of allies.

The PPPs that deal with this particular issue are subject to various limitations that can compromise good governance, understood here as achieving the desired results in the right way (HAWKES, 2008b). From this author's perspective, private partners can interact to drive the government's agenda in such a way as to evade their real responsibilities or divert the focus of attention to potential solutions that run counter to their interests. They can also influence the decisions of government partners, creating an internal environment that inhibits them from making efforts to regulate the private sector in order not to jeopardize the partnership already in place.

Majone's (2006) article on the regulatory state brings together various elements that help to understand the actions of governments. According to the author, this new model creates a paradox which is reflected in the encouragement of privatization and deregulation on the one hand, and the increase in regulatory policies on the other. However, in order to adjust to the needs of the market, the rationality of government intervention combines measures of deregulation and new regulation. The Agreement fits in perfectly with deregulation which, according to this author, means flexible, non-rigid regulation and which is applied on a large scale in the field of social regulation, which includes health.

Although the state, in the era of economic globalization, is subject to constant pressure from the international market, forcing it to make various concessions, Santos (2005) believes that it still has enough power to react and manage its rules in such a way as to make external influences and internal realities compatible. However, everything depends on the real interests that the state defends and the skill and strategies used to make them viable.

The Agreement formalized between the government and the entities representing the food industry demonstrably did not take into account internal realities (obesity epidemic, high consumption of high-calorie and high-salt products, increase in other CNCDs). It has been shaped by elastic measures to reduce sodium and still without effective support from the "educational" work of health institutions to make the population aware of the benefits of this reduction. At first, it seems that it is only health that is at stake, but, in a veiled way, there is also a concern to prevent the market, during the product adjustment phase, from suffering a drop in profits as a result of such measures. Because of this, Stuckler & Nestle (2012) state that any partnership must result in profits for the industries.

Thus, this obvious counterbalance of interests implicitly led to the decision not to address the conflicts of sodium regulation, based on the minimum levels indicated by the diagnosis and proven to be feasible, which is one of the weaknesses of this intervention. It is important to note that, in previous experiences, national industries were forced to enrich their products with nutrients to meet the demands of the health sector, bearing the economic costs of this procedure. Now, the confrontation involves transnational companies and the reduction of unhealthy, low-cost nutrients, which affect the palatability of the products and can interfere with sales.

The effects of the Agreements and Terms of Commitment extend to all health surveillance services, since they carry out the product monitoring activities provided for in those acts. In this way, these acts become a cause for reflection, since they have no legal value for routine health surveillance actions. Compared to the ritual of the practices carried out, these acts symbolize treating the market in a protective manner and delaying the guarantee of the public's right to health. In addition, it sets precedents in the field of health surveillance for regulation to be replaced by "agreement" when it is necessary to deal with controversial issues of health risks, increasing the conflicts inherent in the activity.

The fact that excess nutritional components (saturated fats, sugars and salt) produce health effects (accumulative and long-term) that are different from those caused by the majority of contaminating agents (generally short-term and spread extensively and quickly if the product is globally circulated), should not be a reason for the government to adopt different interventions, as it has always applied compulsory rules to this second group of risks.

Although regulation is usually misunderstood as an unfriendly and authoritarian intervention, it is opportune and necessary when it comes to preventing health risks, including epidemics that spread in society. The absence of international parameters, in the face of global trade, on how to deal with the key nutrients present in food products does not prevent the country from daring to protect the health of the public, nor does it prevent it from holding back by adopting slow, mitigating measures in this field. The government was right to choose the path of argument, of convincing, but it was wrong, at the end of the dialogue, not to establish compulsory rules for reducing sodium and the other nutrients in question.

Another aspect of the fragility of this Agreement is the marked absence of civil society. One of the central aspects of "good governance" in any initiative is the representation and participation in decision-making of those affected by the exercise of power (HAWKES, 2011). However, the forced absence of civil society breaks with the practices that have been inaugurated since the 1988 Constitution, the creation of public spaces for intervention and the expression of participatory democracy. This was a marked absence, insofar as civil society could act as a differentiated member, both to support the government in defending the public interest and the primacy of health issues, and to exert pressure in order to advance negotiations for the approval of rules with fairer targets for the reduction of sodium in food products.

To summarize, rather than representing an advance in food control mechanisms, the Agreement represents political-institutional limitations to the practice of health surveillance, especially in three respects: a) it creates precedents to avoid regulation with the aim of reducing the levels of key nutrients, a fundamental action to protect health; b) it creates situations of internal imbroglio, since there is no way to monitor compliance with nutritional levels, based on this Agreement and, finally, c) it reduces civil society to a vacuum, placing it on the margins of this process of agreeing health measures, to ease tensions and clashes with the productive sector. The active participation of organized civil society is always a reinforcement for achieving greater conquests, including the improvement of the nutritional composition of products by industrial corporations.

6 RISKS AND FOOD REGULATION: VIEWS OF SOCIAL SUBJECTS[31]

6.1 Discursive rationalities: an exercise in interpretation

To introduce the analysis, Foucault's (1982) reflections on the notion of "government" are recalled, not strictly referring to government as an institution, but as a practice, understood as a form of complex exercise of power that aims to *"[....] ensure, by various means, that certain ends can be achieved"* (p.284). To this end, government consists of framing men's conduct through the use of tactical instruments, making them adjust themselves to the rules of governmental rationality and, in this way, making the desired intentions come true. It is in this sense that it can be said that every government aims to achieve self-government on the part of the subjects themselves, through which they freely appropriate (or imagine they do so) the rules of conduct imposed by government power.

The general rationality adopted to address the risks attributed to food and the regulatory mechanisms unleashed by the public sphere to control them is differentiated when it is received and practiced by subjects who, in their respective fields of competence, exert interference and shape its construction, as well as conducting their strategies of influence and moving towards action. With different contributions of symbolic and material capital and social commitments that are not always in tune, they follow specific paths that lead decisively to different processes of understanding.

In line with Foucault's sequence, and later developments in AD, it is stated that the constitution of reality is inseparable from the discursive activity that organizes it (FOUCAULT, 1999) and that, in order to understand it, it is necessary to explore language.

In other words, breaking with its pseudo-transparency and investigating the meaning of its production operations, reconstructing the values of its enunciative markers and the meaning of its alterations in the discontinuous thread of the discourse. However, the result achieved will never represent an encounter with the truth of the facts, because language contains a collection of meanings. It is simply a matter of establishing, using theoretical-methodological tools, an analysis of language-subject-meaning and choosing a path for interpretation (ORLANDI, 2010).

Thus, this chapter presents the analysis of a set of discourses, interweaving voices representing key subjects on the behavior of food risks and the consequences derived

---

31 The techniques of Discourse Analysis and the topology of the Semiotic Square were further developed during working sessions with Prof. Dr. Patrick Dahlet, visiting professor at the Federal University of Minas Gerais.

from them, as well as the operative value of the regulatory strategy adopted by national public institutions.

It's important to note that the speeches were collected between February 26, 2013 and June 6, 2013, during recorded interviews. They are the speeches of subjects belonging almost entirely to three types of sectors[32] - the market, public authorities and civil society - which are approached with their own instruments, hierarchy of values and modes of argumentation. Considering that the marks of orality are not significant for reconstructing the meaning intended by the interlocutors in question, the speeches were transcribed without referring to the syntactic and rhythmic fluctuations characteristic of their anchoring in an oral context. The approach chosen refers to the theoretical and methodological foundations of AD (PÊCHEUX, 2008; ORLANDI, 2010).

From this perspective, on a theoretical level, each textual manifestation is inscribed in a discursive universe that pre-forms what can be said and how this intention to say can be actualized in a given context of social and enunciative interaction. This means that each text (in this case, each interview transcript) can always be understood as a unique realization and irreducible to others (the transcripts of the interviews of civil society subjects differ from those of market subjects, for example), due to the singularity of the discursive activity of particular subjects. However, each text necessarily has generic similarities with others, as it circulates at the same time and in the same field of knowledge (in this case, the discourses on risks and food regulation in Brazil), referring both to the proximity of the contents dealt with and the ways in which they are enunciated.

Discourse is the product of a symbolic system that fuses language and ideology. The former is externalized, while the latter acts in the discourses, acting as the guiding thread of distinctions between them, causing positions and symbolic struggles to erupt. These interests at stake become objective correlations of forces between the different agents, the subjects of enunciation, in order to impose their conception of the world and defend their particular purposes as the expression of the social whole (BOURDIEU, 2009). For this reason, it is understood that discourse not only erects ideological representations, but also has its own rationality that underpins practices associated with rules and thus defines how behaviors should conform - in this case, the relationship between food consumption and health.

32 Only one interview was conducted with a representative of an international organization.

One never says or writes anything in any way and in any situation (DAHLET, 1994). According to Pêcheux (2008), any textual manifestation must therefore be conceived as pre-constructed, because it is configured in advance by a range of conditions of enunciative possibilities, which establish the general frameworks and themes in which it will be able to move in order to be worked on.

The existence of such pre-constructions defines matrix statements that will guide, with varying degrees of conformity according to the socio-enunciative positioning of the interlocutors, the set of texts that organizes the discursive representations of the same object of discourse - in this case, Brazilian society's relationship with food quality.

At a methodological level, the delimitation of matrix enunciations makes it possible to identify, at the same time, the affinities of a text in relation to others (related, in this case, to its inscription within the same globalizing neoliberal discourse) and the Significant Variations resulting from the subjects' unique relationships to the thematizations ordered by the matrix enunciations and to the specific social contexts according to which these matrix regularities are filtered by the speakers.

It is thus determined that all the interviews collected move through an argumentative movement directed by five matrix statements, which have been synthesized as enunciative functions that cut across all the discourses studied:

a) **Essentiality** of food: It is postulated that food is life in essence and this essential vitality of food has been enshrined since the origins of humanity. However, what is in vogue is the essentialist reaffirmation of the identity of food in itself, independent of conditioning, which will always be superficial and incapable of shaking its mythical purity. It is only up to man to achieve a balance in food consumption in order to reach the key to health and life.

b) **Irreversibility of industrialized product consumption:** This enunciative regularity calls into question the economic logic of food processing (products aimed at profit and/or nutritional benefits) and the food product resulting from the technological process, comparing it with the authenticity (real or imagined) of food extracted from nature.

c) **Consumer autonomy:** The individual, under the prism of neoliberal ideology, is autonomous in making their food choices. However, eating is a risky act, so the individual is dependent on the wisdom and experience acquired to be able to protect themselves.

d) **Consumers to (trans)form:** The consumer's capacity for self-defense lies in the information received/transmitted, which acts as the engine for transforming their consciousness, having a direct repercussion on their conduct.

e) **Consenting regulation:** Achieving a healthy product does not only involve legal provisions, but also regulatory governance agreed between the interested parties, reconciling the internalization of market values and balanced nutrition.

It is the variations in the discursive realizations of these matrix statements that will be examined successively below, relating, where possible, the differentiation of their meanings, the changes in their formulations between one set of interviews and another, with the aim of delimiting and interpreting the tensions (the play of agreements and conflicts) that run through the promises of a healthy food product to balance everyone's nutrition. At the end, a summary table (Table 4) will be presented, comparing the matrix statements, postulates and discursive realizations, in the light of the interpretation carried out.

a) ***Essentiality of the food.***

Based on the interviews, the conception of food goes in two directions: firstly, food is part of an imaginary and mythical vision of its historical cycles and its passage through human history. It's a kind of mythification of food, which sees it as a source of energy, protein and life for humanity, as well as being capable of concentrating all virtues. Secondly, food is something inherent to nature, and this character does not disappear, despite the human transformations practiced on it. This leads to a kind of unrealization of the product, which means that it is always assumed to be food, by and for nature, remaining unchanged even when modified by industry.

Thus, subject M1 traces a long history of food in human history, since ancient times, and states that: [...] food is one of the fundamental things in human life. [...] what is vital for health, for the existence of human beings, is food. He also points out that from time immemorial [...] the first manifestation was how to preserve food. [...] the first revolution was fire; the second revolution was the discovery of how to sun-dry the product [...] and he concludes by arguing that industrialization is the extension of the ancient "secrets" of food preservation inherited from antiquity.

In this description, industrialized food is necessarily qualified, because technology is exclusively concerned with rescuing the vital properties mythically attributed to food and preserving them so that it can face the challenges of time. Thus, it is up to the industries to do this competently, since they hold the secrets of preservation that were revealed by the ancients, perfecting food with the dynamics imposed by experience and their expectations.

Subject M3, on the other hand, focused his brief historiographical essay on the cycles or waves of food production, revealing the innovations that have taken place in the food product and concluding that, along the way, there has been a loss of the link with nutrition, which needs to be re-established:

[...] we see the cycles of food in Brazil [...] the first big cycle was pre-war, with *fresh* food, everyone had time [...], they ate at home [...] food for special purposes began to appear in the 60s and 70s [...]; the fourth wave [...] was exactly diet and light [...] and the second phase of this fourth wave [...] when we had a change in the understanding of food - it's much more about nutrition [...] it's a food with a certain calorie content....] and the second phase of this fourth wave [...] when we had a change in our understanding of what food is - it's much more about nutrition, in other words, a food with a certain amount of calories, sodium, protein or fat, may or may not help improve health (M3).

The comparison of these two discourses made by market participants shows a clear contradiction in the image of the food product built up over time: in the first discourse, the integrity of food seems to remain unshaken in the face of transformations in society, while in the second discourse, there is recognition of change, but a reductionist view of food prevails, focusing only on its nutrients.

In the market group, there is an appreciation of food as a vital substance, an almost magical vision of the product's vital essence. However, the difference between the discourses is revealed when M1, in reference to this mythical vision of the benefits of food, exempts the food incorporated into the market from any responsibility for the health problems of the community and the individual: I don't think food does any harm, quite the opposite, I'm disgusted when people say that food is bad for you [...] the most incoherent and ignorant phrase I've ever seen in my life [...] (M1).

This consideration actually expresses the basic ideological operating principle of neoliberalism, in which the market aims exclusively to benefit people in all dimensions of life, but cannot and does not wish to impose such benefits, as it violates its own precepts that decree its free operation and the free will of the individual (DAHLET, 2014). From this perspective, it is up to the individual to decide whether or not to take advantage of the benefits offered by the market and, if not, the responsibility for the disturbances falls on this individual decision, which at the same time proves the logic of free enterprise, the foundation of this current of thought.

This exemption of food from responsibility is reiterated under different arguments, to the point where it becomes an autonomous agent of the action: food is not to blame (M1). The food gives rise to a rhetorical personification, which will allow the food itself to become the agent of the production process, as will be pointed out later, thus erasing the responsibility of the industries themselves.

As the interview progresses, this same subject is affected by the pitfalls of discourse, implicitly recognizing the partial responsibility of industrial processing, but keeping the essentiality of food untouched: Chronic non-communicable diseases [...] the causes [...] are multi-causal - they are due to lack of physical activity; too much food with ingredients [...] and it's not only our industrialized food that contains salt (M1). This formulation comes close to contradicting the previous statement - that the food is not to blame. There is also a counter-discourse, in a very controversial context, in which the sodium in industrialized food is highlighted exclusively and the effects of other nutritional components are erased, which, when present in excess in industrialized food, are equally harmful to health. Furthermore, in this discourse, the subject implicitly wants to mitigate the harmful characteristics of industrialized food by sharing them with food made at home - which also uses excessive amounts of unhealthy ingredients, such as salt.

Therefore, the relationship between food and disease is a point where there are variations between the discourses of the three subjects of the market group and, contrary to what might be inferred, within the market group, uniqueness does not shine through. One of the subjects combines the affirmation of the immemorial value of food with the relativization of its beneficial effects, since he attributes excess weight and obesity as one of the consequences related to the consumption of food, without limiting himself to it: So I don't think it (food) is alone. I think we have a combination, unfortunately, of several factors (M3). From the point of view of this subject, food is not recognized as the isolated protagonist of the food tragedy. Other elements circulate with it, diluting its importance. However, as part of the responsibility is delegated to industrialized food, the subject is sensitive and favourable to the use of the "good regulatory governance" strategy. Another subject shares the image drawn by the first, and dismisses any negative implications of industrialized foods, preferring to treat them in a diluted way, as a "diet", recommending only moderation in consumption: I recommend the diet that you eat everything. [...]

Something that moderates this, but doesn't eliminate chocolate, for example, from the diet [...]. Now what you have to do is .... moderate it. [...] You have to balance your needs (M2).

People linked to public authorities and organized civil society also recognize that food is essential to human life. However, they mention the importance of growing and production conditions in preserving the sanitary condition of food, so that human health can benefit and remain in balance. With this, we can even abstract the question of medicine, if we manage to make food our medicine (S3).

Thus, the equalization of the reference to food as an intrinsic source of health is what emerges from the confrontation of all the discourses, whatever their institutional origin. This leads to an imaginary activation of the primitive properties of food, according to the formulations extracted from the interviews:

[...] food is one of the fundamental things in human life. [Food is vital for health, for the existence of human beings (M1). [...] it is the main axis in a person's health (S1). There is a body of information that points to the centrality of the issue of food, of the human-food binomial on the health conditions of the population (P4).

This consensual discourse - that life cannot do without food - persists as a strategic moral rhetoric. In fact, they are symbolic justifications to cover up the competitive process of the market, which is capable of subjecting food to any conditioning, including those capable of making it harmful to health.

In general, the discourses conveyed by the market, public authorities and organized civil society also align themselves with the centrality of food in health and life: Health depends on food (P6). Food influences health in many ways [...] (P4). [Food is life (S2). [Food is the human being's main fuel (S1). Without disregarding the intrinsic positive power of food, considerations are made about the ability of the food product to automatically absorb the intrinsic qualities of the raw material - food - as mentioned in the speeches of the subjects linked to the market. The discourses flowing from the other two groups of subjects state that only select products can carry positive attributes and effectively benefit health. Otherwise, the successive interaction of "ordinary" products with the body will cause physical and functional dysfunctions in the individual during the course of consumption.

Food occupies a central position that can be positive or negative for people's health (P2). [...] it influences health in many ways, both good and bad. Eating good quality, nutritionally adequate food improves quality of life, the body's functions and, consequently, health is preserved (P4). Food reflects on the body itself. [It leads to illness in many ways (P1).

In everyday life, a healthy life is a social conquest. Struggles, clashes and negotiations were required to force an unequal society to make the right to the basic necessities for human survival equal. Aware of this, one of the members of civil society states: We greatly value the achievement we have had in including the right to adequate and healthy food in the Constitution as part of Article 60, which talks about social rights (S2). It is a matter of cheering and praising the collective effort to include food in the set of social rights in the Brazilian Constitution, since food has been ratified as a universal human right since 196633 and only recently[33 34] , in 2010, was it converted into a social right in Brazil, allowing citizens to claim it from public institutions in situations where it is impossible to realize this right.

For those in civil society, even with the almost unanimous understanding of the central role of food in people's lives, this is still not enough for the government to unleash proposals for solutions to the issue, including a review of the food production system. The solutions to the risks arising from food consumption are being circumvented by alternatives outside the system, such as medicalization, the use of production technologies, which are still controversial, and the use of surgical intervention to reduce weight:

[...] there is no deep understanding in society that food is central and that we all have to engage in this perspective [...]. These biofortification proposals also need to be better analyzed from a nutritional point of view, [...] Brazil continues to release transgenics [...] (S2). [...] I was surprised by a measure from the Ministry of Health, an ordinance that came out on obesity [...] which somehow favors bariatric surgery [...] from the age of sixteen [...] it seems that the Ministry's intention is to take care of obesity through this procedure (S3).

It is a fact that the proximity of interest positions increases the points of similarity between the discourses, as seen in the statements made by the public authorities and

33 The Human Right to Adequate Food (HRAF) was recognized in 1966, after the states parties approved the International Covenant on Economic, Social and Cultural Rights (ICESCR) within the framework of the United Nations (UN, 1966).
34 Constitutional Amendment 64, of February 4, 2010, includes food in Article 60 of the Federal Constitution, which deals with social rights (BRAZIL; PRESIDENCY OF THE REPUBLIC, 2010).

organized civil society. Thus, in the exploration of the food-health binomial, based on a collection of extracts from speeches, several coinciding points stand out. Scientific rationality, with a predominance of biologicist traits, mixed with discreet mentions of food culture and the social sphere, intersect in the discursive formations, evoking food-borne illnesses. A conception dominates, in which the pathological entity has a fluid link with the social, which is reduced to a mere factor, while its condition as a determinant is disregarded. Individuals are singled out as responsible, hiding the other social actors involved in the chain and reversal of morbid processes.

[...] the set of diseases that most affect the Brazilian population are strongly determined, to some degree, by the dietary practices of individuals (P2). The statistics for CNCDs, especially diabetes, cardiovascular diseases and some types of cancer, have implications for food and nutrition (P5). [...] the correlation with obesity, in that it has various consequences. [...] changes in cholesterol, blood pressure [...], to the extent that you manage to adjust your weight and improve your diet, this magically has an impact on these consequences (S3) [...] I think the relationship (diet and nutritional profile) is... quite strong. It's obvious that we have other factors, [...] - environmental factors, sociological factors [...] the type of work people do today; so they become sedentary [...] (S1).

In other parts of the speech, the disease is socially constructed and social institutions - family, school, state - contribute in different ways to its appearance and therefore have responsibilities to assume. The market, camouflaged in advertising, is not made explicit in this part of the speech.

[....] how this obesity was built [...]. This construction [...] has various incentives. Incentives from advertising, which even starts with children in front of the television [...]. So it's built up, often through the omission of the family, often in school activities. [...]. Before the family's omission [...]. But before that, the role of the state, when I talk about publicity, [...], the provision of services, ranging from professionals who are well placed in the public network, in short, to offer, to provide services in this sense to the population (S3).

From a kaleidoscopic viewpoint, food, a practice that involves the consumption of food, is made up of different perspectives: interaction, affection and power added to nutrition. Elements of one of the discourses, full of richness and daring, influenced by a totalizing world view, in which other facets are revealed that are interwoven in the object in question. Consuming food goes beyond the function of nourishment to meet bodily needs. It is an instinctive act, but at the same time a social one, impregnated with affective meanings, capable of both fostering interpersonal interaction and sparking conflicts in the field of power:

Feeding is the sharing of food; it's you collectively feeding yourself. There's a ritual involved in nourishing yourself and nourishing a group of people [...]. That's why food is very symbolic. It (food) is ceasing to be seen as a sacred element and is very much bent by a logic of consumption and expressions of power (P1).

The consumer market has articulated the logic of pleasure with that of desire. The first sensation is necessarily meant to work for a short period of time, while in the second, the rule is to always remain active and incomplete, remaining open to new opportunities that the market in its dynamism will make available. The food product actively participates in this game of marketing seduction and, in general, the score points to the consumer as the loser - the one who loses health and gains illness and anguish, due to the biological and material limits to consumption.

This consumerist logic leads to obesity, not just of the body, but obesity of thought, of the senses. Consumerism is an expression of today's society and it is very much in dialogue with drug addiction, not least because it means the search for immediate, flashy pleasure (P1).

As shown above, we can see the hallmarks of the distinction between the discourses of public authorities and civil society and those of the market, which can be summarized in three main points:

a) the interconnection between food and disease, which results from a mismatched relationship between the individual and the consumption of industrialized food, situated in a context of a society whose gears are permissive for production. At the same time, it is restrictive for individuals. They have to make a continuous effort to properly select what they eat and move their bodies regularly in order to maintain their health, as illustrated below:

The obesity epidemic is related to the consumption of industrialized foods" (P4). Obesity and overweight have two fundamental components: a sedentary lifestyle, lack of regular exercise, and diet (P5). [...] the percentage of obesity today is a pathology that is getting much worse in the population. This is due to excessive consumption of concentrated foods or foods with a high concentration of sodium, fats in general [...] (P6).

b) a broad view of the problems affecting food, which involve both the nutrients in its composition and the inputs used in its production (agrotoxins) and the technology applied to them (transgenic foods): [...] the concern about food has grown a lot with chemical inputs, agrotoxins and the release of transgenics (S2).

c) the food, or rather the food product, internalizes a "good/bad" typology for health, eliminating the "naturalistic conception of food". This is the counterpoint to those who speak on behalf of the market: [...] food doesn't do any harm. I think that's the most incoherent and ignorant sentence I've ever seen in my life (M1). The harmful character attributed to food goes against the ideas conveyed by the market world, which perceives its product as the result of infallible health safety technology, overcoming flaws, risks or deformations: The adoption of these foods is undoubtedly closely linked to the damage done to health today - the amount of sugar, salt [...] (P5).

Finally, it is worth highlighting the widespread use of the term "food" to disguise the food product; a term that is transposed to any type of edible goods, without even naming as products those that are subjected to a high degree of artificialization and can only be identified as such before consumption, exclusively by the aromas exhaled that simulate those of nature, and which lead individuals to associate them with the food imaginary.

b) Irreversibility of consumption of the industrialized product.

The food product fits into the hegemonic lifestyle, bringing together special characteristics such as being practical, quick and having disposable packaging, meeting the expectations of urbanites, whose rule is to have little time to devote to food. It also meets the logic of the consumerist economy of producing ephemeral desires and insatiable needs, allowing for constant innovation and substitution of products. Considering the context of urbanization, the three groups of subjects agree on the irreversibility of industrialized product consumption in urbanized society:

The trend towards industrialized food is really increasing, not least because of work; in short, we eat very little lunch at home and consume industrialized food (P3). Processed food is interwoven into modern life. [...] people don't have time to prepare food [...] (P4). Food industries are now a necessity for the modern population, as eating out is one of today's characteristics (P6). Industrialized food is a necessity (M2). [...] modern life wouldn't exist if it weren't for industrialized food (M1). [...] the share of processed food in today's society is growing (S1).

In the case of the market, the definitive conquest of the food product in the social space refers to two fundamental representations: the first consists of the general affirmation of its indispensable role for humanity, [...] industrialized food is a necessity [...]. [...] without industry we wouldn't be able to feed everyone, so there is a need for the industrialization of food (M2).] without industry we wouldn't be able to feed everyone, so there is a need for the industrialization of food (M2); the second states that industrialized food is idealized as a symbol of the avant-garde; it is confused with modernity itself, not just because it is "food in itself", but because it has broken new ground, acting as one of the driving forces behind female freedom and human longevity. Thus, [...] there would be no modern life if it weren't for industrialized food. Women wouldn't leave the house because they'd have to prepare food for their children (M1).

From the point of view of one of the subjects linked to the market, the application of technology in the food production sector is a measure of quality, as it enhances its nutritional aspects and increases its shelf life, as well as guaranteeing the health safety of the product. For people in this sector, nothing is beyond their control and nothing is like other experiences in industrial practice; and they admit that negative externalities are a possibility in production activity. Thus, dysfunctions or damage to health escape the world of industrialized food:

[...] processing - processing means [...] preparing to preserve the food for as long as possible [...] to present it to the consumer in a more suitable way, in an environment in which it can be consumed *healthily* and with the guarantee that it won't harm them (M1).

It can be seen in the above excerpt that, in the production-consumption relationship, the industry projects itself as an agent that reacts to the needs of the consumer; it goes out of its way to seek innovations and adjustments in order to make products to meet the consumer's needs. In this discourse, the roles are reversed: the consumer is the one who creates needs and the industry merely meets them. A "passivity" that is incompatible with its ability to disseminate the product, generate needs and insist on successful sales.

The statements made by public authorities and civil society go against the grain of those made by market players, and undo the ideal of purity of food products by placing them in the current context. In the sum of the broken statements, diseases originate within the food market itself, which is in charge of manufacturing food products and which behaves as an agent carrying two simultaneous functions: the operative one of causing diseases and the symbolic one of exterminating food traditions:

The obesity pandemic is linked to the market. [...] there are foods that are addictive - soft drinks are addictive; sugar is addictive (P1). The food has to be harmless to the consumer

[...] and it has to meet the consumer's habits (P3). Our dietary pattern is turning a lot towards over-processed foods that have a lot of chemical components in their composition [...], as well as sodium, all the sweeteners, as well as all the other additives [...] I wouldn't know how to explain the illnesses [...] (S2).

For one of the interviewees, linked to the market group that treats the food product as excellence, it is implicit that no harm will be done to the consumer by this product. It personalizes the food and naturalizes its qualities, anchoring it in the resources of nature [...] our raw material grows by the hand of the land (M1), with industry unable to surpass the land in terms of production capacity. It is the food itself and the land that dictate the quality of the food, and so he is emphatic in contesting any slander directed at the quality of the product: [...] there is no point in diminishing our product. They won't get fat off our product, they'll get fat off everything else (M1).

However, despite the majority of interests shared within the market group, two subjects differ in their understanding of the behavior of food products in terms of quality. For them, the differences in the quality of food products are real and are reflected in the content and price: a) products that contain an excess of certain key ingredients (sugar and fat) in their formulation are harmful to health and have lower prices; b) improving the nutritional profile of products is associated with higher prices:

[...] products with a lot of sugar, excess fat, there wasn't so much concern about these characteristics until recently (M3). The industry [...] is putting more nutritious products on the market. Now it depends on the social class that can afford it. The better off people are, the more they will seek out this type of product. So, if you had a greater volume of production, you could reduce it, but it's already more expensive on its own (M2).

From these considerations, it becomes clear that the food market responds to the stratification of society, creating qualitatively differentiated product lines for social classes ranked by purchasing power. These socially marked production lines are divided into food products with lower nutritional quality and more affordable prices, which lead to a greater negative impact on health, exposing the population in the lower socio-economic strata to risks. On the other hand, those products with a nutritional profile close to the precepts of what is healthy, and which are more expensive, are aimed at a special audience, with higher purchasing power and the ability to afford them. It can be seen that food products, like any other good with a

They have symbolic value and are characterized by distinctions (BOURDIEU, 2011). Thus, the type of food consumption externalizes and makes it possible to identify the differentiated position of individuals in the social structure.

Committed to the collective interest, the civil society interviewees unveil the masks associated with these key nutrients, covered up by the industries. These nutrients, added to additives and incorporated into the product's formulation, behave like real tricks used by the industry to win over and retain consumer loyalty. These artifices bring the aroma and taste of the manufactured product closer to that of natural food, as well as making it attractive in terms of price and presentation:

Fat and sugar bring flavor to food. So, if you want to captivate an audience so that they consume that food, the side of the person designing the food will say: load up on salt; load up on sugar and load up on fat [...]. In addition to flavorings, artificial things added to enhance aroma and taste; sugar, fat and salt are elements that captivate the consumer's taste; they are cheap ingredients (S1). Because brands are proliferating, including the cheapening of these over-processed products, for example [...] these little biscuits, these things that even look like..., I don't know, chips (S2).

For two members of civil society, the risks posed by these key nutrients deserve to be warned about on food labels: Our regulations are still very tenuous, because even today there is debate about whether these foods are excessively fatty or not, and warnings need to be put on labels so that they can be consumed thoughtfully, because I'm in favor (P6).

One of them suggests that we could comply with the warnings applied to regulate traffic, considering that a set of mandatory labeling information for food products is insufficient to keep the consumer under constant attention. Thus, the use of certain universal illuminated signs, already introjected by individuals, is always convenient to warn the population against numerous risks and dangers, in order to establish control and protection, such as: [...] the nutritional traffic light adopted in some places in Europe, which signals if a certain food is too rich in a nutrient. So this is interesting from an information point of view (S1).

Thus, adapting the logic of traffic lights to the nutritional field would allow consumers to visualize the classification of foods in terms of the content of certain nutrients. This is a form of risk communication that is quick to see and easy to understand. However, it is the government, due to its regulatory role, that has to become aware of this proposal and make it operational, or some other proposal that meets these needs.

When it comes to the commercial quality of products, the emphatic phrase of one of the market participants is at odds with the previous comment: Nobody gets to be the second largest food producer in the world and export industrialized products, processed products, semi-processed products to 114 countries [...]. We don't talk about food without nutritional quality, just as we talk about quality (M1).

From the point of view of the market, the full satisfaction of product quality is demonstrated by commercial expansion. Here, quality becomes the expansion of the product in foreign trade. It is with a similar type of argument, the international acceptance of the product, that the aim is to empty the limited spaces of those who believe in and mobilize to justify the use of warnings and other measures to regulate the consumption of food products.

However, one of the market players positions the food industry as an integral part of society as a whole, and therefore as a bearer of responsibility towards society. For him, the food industry, out of prudence, should not distance itself from, or even deny, the ills of the social world, especially when the food product is involved in them. Paying attention to corrective measures can be a useful strategy to remain stable or expand the market: I think that industries do have a very big responsibility to worry about what is on offer and what kind of characteristics the product should have. [...] the role of the industry is to be connected to this new epidemiological situation (M3).

From the point of view of civil society, the pressure exerted on the industry is demanding a response from it, but the reaction is timid, aimed at expanding the portfolio of differentiated products, but leaving the nutritional composition of the vast majority of products untouched. It is known that reversing the nutritional quality of these foods entails costs, due to the substitution of ingredients with others of higher nutritional quality, which are relatively more expensive, consequently causing losses in company profits, which are growing at an excessive rate.

[...] there is pressure for it (the industry) to improve this quality [...] at the speed that would be necessary. [...] There's more emphasis on marketing, appeals that you have on the packaging [...] that it's *light*, that it's *diet* [...] to gain a share of the market [...] a timid stance. [...] The concern of [...] every industry, every business is to make a profit. [...] to improve food you need to invest in technology and development [...] spending money is what nobody wants (S1).

It can also be seen in this statement that it is these appeals, imported from the American food standard (*diet* and *light*), aimed at a certain section of the population, which give the product a sense of effectiveness and social distinction, as mentioned above.

Sales of industrialized food products are mobilized by a sophisticated and convincing commercial and advertising apparatus, which violates the traditional values of local food culture and induces Brazilians to change their preferences in favour of industrialized products: The POF and PNAD surveys show, for example, [...] the growth in the consumption of filled cookies and soft drinks is absurd! And at the same time, we have a big reduction in Brazil in the consumption of rice, beans, fruit and vegetables [...] (S2).

What was once supposition is now proven fact. The effects of the food industry's activities, which are not restricted to Brazil, but are spreading throughout the world, have already taken effect, in terms of standardizing the habits and consumption practices of the earth's inhabitants; imposing a style of behaviour; rationalizing production costs; and exorbitantly increasing their profits.

If the market respects the consumer, it respects their eating habits, because they are eating habits filtered by the interests of the market. The concern about breaking this link and losing sales is the controversy faced by the production sector and revealed in the speech of its representative: [...] Brazilians are used to eating more salty food [...]. So if you remove too much (salt), it will become tasteless and this product will stop being sold in the end (M2).

For the market, changing the product formula should not affect commercial profits. It is therefore essential that the government explains to the public the importance of changing the composition of products, so that it is appreciated by the public, avoiding rejection of products and a drop in sales. This is because reducing the sodium content has an impact on the sensory quality of the food product: The industry is also looking; it's just that society, the government itself, has to play its part, which is to clarify (M2). The market argues that the government, in return for the industries' efforts to reformulate food products, should educate the public to accept these "reformulated" products, as this is a way of protecting the market.

However, when it comes to the government guiding the market itself, i.e. disciplining unhealthy food products, so that they are in line with public policy to prevent obesity and other CNCDs, the representative of this segment makes it implicit, at various points in his speech, that there is no justification for government interference in the industry's business, since the products are suitable: [....] I don't think that food is killing as many people as they are saying. It's much more scaremongering [...]. How long have you not heard [...] scandals [...] someone died or someone got sick because of industrialized products (M1).

When the subject of food advertising came up, several speeches by people linked to public power and organized civil society defended the need for regulation and denounced the pressures of the production sectors on the government:

[...] food education [...] can have several fronts [...] it can be present in restricting the advertising of certain foods [...] (S1). Food advertising also needs to be better regulated; this principle of adequate and healthy food should be the focus (S2). In the case of food advertising, the government has suffered and been hampered by the actions of the industry itself" (P6). There is also concern about the level of food advertising that is completely unregulated in the country, of foods that are harmful to health and very much aimed at children (P1). A diet that is determined by the market and with a lack of regulation, including of advertising. The consumption of industrialized food is closely linked to the world of marketing and advertising, which induces inappropriate eating habits (P5).

The concern with advertising lies in the stimulation of consumption and the resulting change in traditional healthy eating habits, which leads to disease. By adhering to a dietary practice imposed by the market, individuals promote the strengthening of this market and, at the same time, damage their health and their food culture. The speeches show the industry's interference in the handling of public affairs and the government's retreat, as happened with the rules governing food advertising aimed at children. After its publication, the approved regulation suffered numerous criticisms from opponents, culminating in its suspension by judicial measures brought by the industry and media companies.

The relationship between the advertising of unhealthy food products and *the* repercussions on health has been reinforced for some time, and this intervention has the backing of the Federal Constitution of 1988, in its article 227, which states: *It is the duty of the family, society and the state to ensure children and adolescents, with absolute priority, the right to life, health [...].* The issue is not technical, but political, and the obstacles lie within the body of parliamentarians in the National Congress, who do not respect the Constitution. This is because they are unwilling to confront the economic forces, since these serve as a springboard for many of them to be elected as formal representatives of the people; but, in fact, what they defend are the interests of the productive sector.

[...] this Congress needs, for the protection of our population, to restrict advertising, at least in the hours when children are most vulnerable and, at the same time, to follow what the Constitution recommends. Advertising and marketing play a very important role and, behind this, there is a whole business community, that is, an economic force, which has political power, because our model is more private than public funding and, therefore, around 200 companies practically fund campaigns in Brazil [...]. These companies are the ones who do the advertising and who support the media, which are concentrated in the hands of a few and their profits depend on it - and therein lies the difficulty, the *lobbies* in Congress to influence MPs or intimidate them if they go against them. [...] It's something of a political struggle here in parliament, we are prioritizing and recognizing the political difficulties of approving [...] (P5).

The discourses analyzed highlight the contradictions surrounding food products which, despite the advantages they generate, and engendered by the technological innovations of modernity - such as comfort and durability - are capable of causing a delayed evil with constant consumption driven by advertising, leaving consumers fragile - especially those who are socially vulnerable.

c) Consumer autonomy

The neoliberal spirit that drives contemporary society overburdens the individual with responsibilities towards their body, in order to keep it intact and fit to act as a workforce. The individual is urged to create self-protection mechanisms against risks that he did not produce; to keep an eye on technical information in order to practice self-care; to aim for health integrity; and to engage in self-control in order to keep his body regulated (PETERSEN & LUPTON, 2000). In short, the conditions of well-being and health are the responsibility of the individual, and any deviation in behavior will mean failure, non-commitment and illness, which they will have to bear themselves.

These premises give shape to the speeches coming from market representatives, whose focus is unanimously on blaming the consumer for the lack of brakes on food intake, for not knowing how to balance their diet, for sedentary lifestyles and for the diseases they contract. The excerpts from speeches on the relationship between the obesity pandemic and food serve as an illustration:

[...] if you eat 2000 calories and burn 1000 calories, you'll become obese (M1). [...] the increase in sedentary lifestyles [...] people becoming more and more complacent [...] they don't exercise or do less physical activity. It's not just food (M3). If you don't eat a moderate diet, you can become obese [...] (M2).

Another interviewee in the group, when talking about this issue, prefers to eliminate the figure of the human agent, The excess is the great enemy (M1), and replace the individual responsible with a substantial entity "the excess" that takes over human decisions. In this way, the involvement of industrial activity is neutralized and the responsibility of the product is erased. Here, the statement shifts to moral judgment, as if everyone should achieve balance in the face of everyday events.

In a continuation of this interviewee's speech, there is the intersection of the economic and religious discursive formations, when the interviewee relies on the leading infractions that conform to the precepts of the Christian era. In his explanation, the man who doesn't cultivate his own spiritual virtues becomes a sinner and the blame and the burden of punishment fall solely on him; thus, he reiterates individual responsibility in the face of obesity: [...who is to blame for overeating and its consequences is the consumer himself - it is he who consumes - it is the human being who, in greed, greed, gluttony, overdoes what he does or doesn't prepare himself properly, he who is to blame (M1).

In a timely manner, the use of Christian individualist interdiscourse underpins two justifications: a) the imperfection of man, who is unable to self-impose limits on his own intake and; b) the exclusion of strategic elements that influence individual behavior from the explanatory framework: industry, which produces and stimulates food consumption, and the government, which imposes rules on production-consumption.

The controversy facing the consumption of food products is seen as analogous to that previously faced by the consumption of alcoholic beverages. In both situations, excess is harmful to health. The use of food advertising with consumer warnings can be positive, but without the need to ban or suspend advertising, similar to what is done to limit the consumption of alcoholic beverages. In an implicit way, one of the discourses of the subjects linked to the market, based on the Brazilian epidemiological situation, simulates an alternative of advertising, through commercial vehicles, a warning to avoid excessive consumption of these products and contain the adverse effects on health. In this way, he adapts the phrase that is already used in advertising for alcoholic drinks to food products: Eat in moderation (M2). However, he always makes it clear that this is the consumer's responsibility.

However, without detracting from the sensitivity of this idea, this statement also conceals three advantages that could benefit the market: it avoids the banning of food products that pose a greater risk to health; it rescues injunctions already ingrained in common sense in advertisements against alcohol and smoking; and it demonstrates that the industry is committed to the consumer and is concerned about their well-being and the health of the community.

This *slogan* also implies the unspoken: the evidence of individuals' lack of control over eating and the need to warn them to re-establish self-control, since the solution depends exclusively on them. In this way, the debate is transferred from the socio-political field to the moral field, exempting the industries from any implications and allowing the food trade to continue to flourish without limits, since it becomes the individual's sole responsibility to control what and how much they consume.

In a certain situation, elements of the market's discourse coincide with those of the public authorities, reinforcing that it is the wrong practices of individuals that cause illness:

[...] just as obesity was constructed, it must be deconstructed in the same process. [...] it's not through starvation, it's not through a diet that doesn't meet the person's needs, but through a process of changing habits" (S3). Chronic non-communicable diseases [...] are multi-causal [...] lack of physical activity, too much food with ingredients, and it's not just our industrialized food that contains salt (M1).

However, when these statements are analyzed together, on the one hand there is the figure, explicit or not, of the incapable subject who needs self-transformation in order to control the disease and, on the other, the product summarized as a mere causal factor, obscured in the articulated web that operates in the social world.

Consumer is the reference that stands out in the market. However, depending on the speaker's connection, in certain pronouncements, it is replaced by individual, citizen or aggregate to the collective, in terms of population. In general, the discursive formations of public authorities and civil society mention citizens or the population - to whom their actions are directed. For them, the population does not behave like an amorphous mass when faced with food issues that directly affect their lives and health, and information is seen as the leaven that can raise their awareness of the risks:

[...] but the population has had a lot of encouragement and has become aware, although not to the desired extent [...] of the importance of food in a person's life (S3). There is a reasonable sample who have more access to information and are more sensitive, but they don't always act in practice (P5). The main approach to containing this epidemic is risk communication; making consumers aware of the importance of eating healthier food [...]

(P4).

For one of the interlocutors, there is still the conviction that there are external stimuli that give the collective the impetus to mobilize and thus make a process of reflection, reaction and revision of thinking and acting mature.

Eating is no longer an instinctive act to satisfy biological and emotional needs. Nowadays, knowing how to eat properly requires the mastery of rational knowledge and skills to make the right choice and establish a regulated consumption of food. This involves a regulated freedom, a historically acquired cultural heritage and particular conditions of existence, which can lead to a dietary practice guided by a purely dietary rationality, which encourages disciplining the body to avoid the onset of disease: I don't think food alone solves anything. It can reduce; if the person doesn't know how to eat, they'll overeat and it'll be the same [...] (M3). It should also be added that learning to eat, although cultural, is dynamized and shaped by social influences. Thus, the taste and preference for industrialized products - which are considered harmful to health - are socially acquired through repetition of experience, and are largely fostered by the stimuli of commercial advertising.

Even if the disguise covering certain types of food product, which hides the harm they can cause to health, is removed and the need for their intrinsic modification is reaffirmed, the other part of the responsibility falls on the individual: they must commit to moving their body systematically. Thus, from this individual's point of view, the solution lies: I think that food, with a reduction in these key nutrient issues, and an ever-increasing practice of physical activity are going to be two fundamental links (M3). In search of solutions to widespread overweight, the analysis of a complex sociocultural phenomenon - food consumption - is simplified, transporting it to a reduced and superficial context as a form of health defense.

Still from the market's perspective, consumers are not sufficiently qualified to understand the content of labels, the means by which the industry makes information about the product on offer transparent: [...] Reading labels is not normal in this country. We're wrong to say that everyone reads labels. Many still read the date and expiry date of the product (M2). It is important to point out here that providing information on product labels is not just a legal requirement. It is also an expression of the right to information, and a means of communicating the identity and quality characteristics of the product, to make it easier to compare them and guide the choice. This is technical information that has not yet become popular enough to be understood and valued by the general public, with the exception of the expiry date, which is self-explanatory.

In addition, it is necessary to invest in forms of labeling communication that use clear, accessible language and allow messages to be easily identified, such as the nutritional traffic light. Valuing the right to information requires the decoding of technical messages, enabling everyone to master them, and adjusted to a life context in which the time dedicated to reading product labels is increasingly scarce.

For market players, the issue is not the food products themselves, but the consumer who, due to their intellectual and material limitations, is unable to enjoy a food product with a bivalent character, which has the properties of feeding and nourishing at the same time:

[There are people who are concerned, people who read, people who understand, but let's not forget that the vast majority of Brazilians work to eat. So, with all due respect, they want to eat first; then they'll worry about what to eat - this is the second phase (M2). [...] consumer misinformation about what the product actually offers (M3).

According to market discourse, the problem lies with the mass of consumers, whose profile is one of incompetence, ignorance and misinformation, and whose interest in food is still primarily aimed at satisfying primary needs, without establishing technical criteria for their selection. As a result, consumers remain the weakest link in the chain; they have negative attributes that make it impossible for them to choose food products with a healthy nutritional profile, either because they are uninformed or because their purchasing power is restricted. For the public authorities and organized civil society, there is a lack of information on the part of consumers, which limits their awareness of what an adequate diet consists of.

In the play of discourses between different subjects, the position of the consumer in the face of food risks can be summarized as either victim or culprit. In the first case, it is characterized by poor qualifications and a lack of civic awareness that subjugates them to the impositions of the market and, in the second, by their incompetence in limiting their self-consumption, reading the technical information on product labels correctly and adopting a less sedentary lifestyle.

d) Consumer to (trans)form

Although without clarifying the precise meaning given to "education", it is mentioned by several people as one of the relevant intervention measures aimed at the population. It remains to be seen whether this proposed education actually involves an exchange of knowledge that seeks to stimulate people's ability to reflect on reality, or whether it is simply a transfer of information, with no commitment to any kind of change.

Today, anyone walks into a supermarket and sees a shelf with hundreds of options and you're not going to ban any of them. The way to tackle this is with information, guidance, education, so to speak, in a bigger, broader way - food education (S1). We are now running a campaign aimed at eating out. [...]. The main focus is on encouraging healthy eating, in educational practices, in a preventive approach [...] (S3).

This statement contains three types of instruction - education, information and guidance - aimed at the population on the best way to eat, which will be discussed below.

Education, among these modalities, is considered the only tool that can counteract marketing strategies and prevent the unbridled force of inducement to buy from dominating the individual and turning consumption into an unconscious act. Education enables the individual to reflect and analyze the facts in their critical dimension. However, education must be conceived as a reflexive process of learning knowledge and internalizing common norms, rules and values. And, in this way, enabling the individual to recognize their role as a social being and as a member of a society that presupposes coexistence with others. In this sense, successful education doesn't provide solutions, but leads the subject to question practices. Enlightened by Freire's (2010) political-ideological conception, education in this context should be a means of awakening concerns about the problem of food risks and developing a consciously critical attitude towards it, as advocated by this democratic pedagogical practice.

As far as the information modality is concerned, it involves introducing knowledge in an automated way, without a process of reflection. It is the unilateral transfer of information - and the obtaining of mechanical responses to the commands elicited by this information. Orientation, on the other hand, if it is not based on a dialogic and transformative relationship, can result in similar outcomes to information.

The market discourse also evokes "education" in order to reorient the population in terms of food consumption practices. Don't think that you can do without fat; you'll have to eat a little fat, but you'll have to eat it. So we're going to have to use education in some way so that there's no more than that (M1). The use of "we" indicates that society as a whole is responsible, including the market. However, in the course of this subject's speech, the "we" is reduced to the government and the market is exempt from this responsibility: The government is making the biggest mistake in history, looking only at industrialized products and not focusing on the rest and we are not the whole; we are a part. The government has to educate (M1).

This discourse looks at education from a reductionist perspective. Educating is not just about articulating the causal links of a given phenomenon. It is above all to understand it critically; it is the search for the authenticity of the phenomenon "risks-food-disease", which will lead to the development of critical awareness (FREIRE, 2010). In the speeches mentioned above, the concept of education is reduced to the dimension of providing information, as if this were enough. There also seems to be an understanding that the process of accumulating information could generate awareness and change behavior.

Those involved in civil society, public authorities and international organizations are unanimous on the idea of empowering the population. For them, this is an alternative to recovering and valuing the traditional, healthy food that has been lost:

I think we need to increasingly encourage, stimulate and develop food and nutrition education processes so that people are more empowered to make choices (OI). This movement to improve the nutritional quality of food [...] can't just come from the government, it needs the engagement of organized civil society too [...] (P4). Perhaps nowadays we can say [...] that there is a nascent concern, [...] that I hope this awareness of food will grow (S2).

In this sense, the Food and Nutrition Education Reference Framework - EAN[35] was created with the aim of being a fundamental strategy for promoting healthy eating practices and preventing and controlling food and nutrition problems (BRASIL; MDS, 2012b). Based on an emancipatory perspective, its purpose goes beyond the act of making the individual an active and autonomous being in terms of food choices and practices, and encompasses their ability to (re)interpret the world and themselves, in other words, to direct and transform their own lives. This means empowerment.

It is interesting to note that the subjects realize that tackling the issue of food risks is not restricted to the field of health and education; it also invades social structures, with emphasis on the way production-consumption is organized, in order to make it possible

35 The Food and Nutrition Education Reference Framework for Public Policies, in the context of realizing the Human Right to Adequate Food and guaranteeing Food and Nutrition Security, is a field of knowledge and practice that is continuous and permanent, transdisciplinary, intersectoral and multi-professional and which aims to promote the autonomous and voluntary practice of healthy eating habits (BRASIL; MDS, 2012b). It is a field of action that covers aspects related to food, feeding and nutrition, as well as processes related to the production system.

to re-establish and consolidate a health-based food practice.

[...] to respond to obesity, but the real fight against the social and environmental determinants of obesity takes place in other spaces, including the model of food production and distribution, social programs, education, direct consumer communication, a whole range of other agendas. Tackling obesity requires an intersectoral response (P2).

However, in its structuring principles, the EAN proposes rescuing the different facets of the food phenomenon, by considering an integrated approach to the food system, social, environmental and economic sustainability, valuing local food culture, promoting self-care and the autonomy of individuals, among other aspects. According to this Reference Framework, EAN involves broad and transdisciplinary knowledge, coupled with intersectoral and multi-professional practice, to promote autonomy and voluntariness in adopting healthy eating habits (BRASIL; MDS, 2012).

Even so, promoting EAN as an institutionalized practice does not exempt the state from its duty to curb the excesses committed by the market and which have repercussions on social life, especially on the most vulnerable group of the population. This includes children, who are intellectually immature individuals and therefore still powerless to make their own choices and criticize the stimuli they receive.

It is true that initiatives in the field of social policies in Brazil have had a positive economic effect on the poorest sections of the population, with positive repercussions on access to food. With regard to poverty reduction, it can be seen that the implementation of the Zero Hunger Program, starting in 2003, managed to reduce the poverty rate of the Brazilian population from 28.1% to 15.4% in 2009 (DEL GROSSI, 2010). This contributed positively to the improvement in the nutritional status of children aged zero to five years old in families assisted by the Bolsa Familia Program between 2008 and 2012 (BRASIL; MDS; MS, 2014).

However, the material advancement of this social group, reflected in their progressive participation in the consumer market for different goods, was also seen in the increase in consumption of different industrialized food products. This phenomenon can be considered predictable, due to pent-up demand, built up over long periods of exposure to consumer incentives, but restricted by financial conditions. In addition, food companies have developed specific *marketing* strategies, types of packaging and forms of retail to capture the millions of families who have increased their income through social policies.

Along the way, health education in general and food and nutrition education in particular have continued at their traditional pace and have had little (if any) dialogue with this new reality for families:

Today, there is a whole social change, [...] which brings a certain risk to this awareness that... the guy who only ate rice and beans and manioc flour and, from time to time, an egg; it's good that he can eat other things. But [...] he prefers, then, from the point of view of social *status* - which is legitimate [...] to eat hamburgers, [...] or sausages, or [...] noodles [...]. They can [...] eat more, but not always better (S1).

This comment is consistent with the tendency to choose industrialized products with low nutritional quality, which is evident among the poorest part of the population, according to the latest data from the POF 2008/2009 (BRASIL; IBGE, 2010). This association between dietary pattern and *status* is well-founded, since *status* is defined more by symbolic traits than by actual economic differences (BOURDIEU, 2011). In this way, consuming certain food products that were previously excluded from the diet leads, in the imagination of poor individuals, to social ascension through the representation that these products embody, and which is disseminated in their advertisements. A similar situation was observed with families benefiting from the Bolsa Familia Program: once their basic food needs have been met, they turn to both healthy foods (fruit, vegetables and legumes) and industrialized products with a high energy density and low nutritional value (IBASE, 2008).

In general, the specific discussion of food quality remains far from the agenda of social movements. Few organizations dedicate themselves to the issue and turn it into a platform for struggle and permanent attention. However, according to one of the representatives of a civil society organization, with the opening up of movements to discussion on the issue of "defending food sovereignty" in recent years, the expectation is that concern about the quality of food will be raised: It's interesting that there is a mobilization of many social movements for food sovereignty; I think that the fact that movements are now incorporating the defence of food sovereignty among their causes brings this vision of the food we eat closer (S2).

The lack of knowledge about the complexity of the food-health binomial currently faced by society is not the exclusive privilege of lay people; it also occurs in academic circles, especially affecting health professionals whose duties include the prevention and treatment of diseases, including those related to inadequate food consumption.

Expanding the knowledge of health professionals - both about the complexity of contemporary food processes, but also in participatory education approaches - is one of the current challenges, including in the training of nutritionists (RECINE; MORTOZA, 2013). These are the paths pointed out by the public authorities as a means of curbing obesity:

[...] the population has the right to know the epidemiological profile so that they can direct prevention campaigns. If you make the population aware of the quality of food, not just in advertising campaigns, but in the doctor's training about being overweight, having a different diet, and referring the patient to a nutritionist (P1).

In the field of food, the demands coming from social forces - the market and society - which are sent to the government to be managed, do not always result in decisions in which collective interests prevail over private ones, either for internal reasons or because of weaknesses in the pressure from society as a whole. In this sense, and without naming the agent responsible for mobilizing society - but excluding the government from the commitment to be the leader - individuals linked to public power point out in their discourse that without the strength of citizens who are sensitive to the conflicts over food and health, the government is unable to make the necessary changes in this field happen:

[...] it's important that this food issue isn't concentrated in the space of organized civil society alone, citizens need to take on this reflection, because I don't think we have the strength to move the agenda (P2). The critical mass is small [...] but if other links in society take up this policy, we will succeed very quickly (P4).

It's true that the market's inductive attitude to winning over consumers makes use of the essential trait of the human being: that of being a subject with the potential to become conscious and autonomous of their own actions. Now, he - the human being - is the object of manipulation by the market, which subtly decides for him what is pleasurable to eat, where and how to eat, making him disconnect from the fundamental issues surrounding the act of feeding and nourishing oneself. In this sense, one of the individuals linked to the public authorities calls for the consumer to be provided with information, in order to recover the symbolic values intrinsic to human nature, which have been dampened by market interference: We need to free the human being inside each consumer, so that the human being is not diminished and the condition of the consumer is increased, so that as much information as possible is available about the food that is provided in public spaces (P1). However, as discussed above, it is not information that transforms, but information inserted into a context of education as a critical and participatory process.

For some members of the public, Brazilian civil society is characterized by a lack of historical experience in the struggle for citizenship rights. As a result, when it comes to dealing with the effects of the relationship between food and health, the role it assumes is quite ambivalent in the discourses formulated. Despite recognizing the weakness of civil society, which means that it continues to depend on support and information from the state in order to understand and become aware of the problems that affect it, its action is essential in order to put pressure on the state when it comes to managing conflicts involving food quality. This is because they are a social force capable of opposing others and fighting to make collective health interests a reality.

Civil society is at a standstill, it doesn't have the quality of struggle that the country needs (P6). [...] it's important that this food issue isn't concentrated in the space of organized civil society alone, citizens need to take on this reflection, because I don't think we have the strength to move this agenda (P2). The role of the state is not to replace popular organization, [...] but to foster it, to raise the level of awareness, to raise the level of information (P1).

However, there are real and historical difficulties that inhibit the organization of society, as the following comments point out. The subject of public power points out that the successive experiences of social oppression that the Brazilian people have lived through in their history have imprinted fear, disbelief and the inability to organize themselves to fight for the interests of the whole on the collective unconscious, which hinders or delays the strengthening of social movements and the meeting of demands of collective interest:

[...] there are organized segments that do, but the vast majority are not prepared. [...] Given our history - colonialism, slavery and dictatorship - pieces of which are still present today, we don't have a civil society that is up to the demands of citizenship in this country, marked by "big houses and slave quarters" (P1).

Obviously, the situations of oppression and intimidation imposed on the majority of the population by the Brazilian elite, coupled with generalized impoverishment and a lack of education in the broad sense, which have persisted throughout the country's economic and social development, have contributed to the formation of the Brazilian people with such a fighting profile. Thus, providing this population with an educational tool that can give them full autonomy to make choices in the area of food and, consequently, to oppose the dictatorship of the market, is one of the functions of the state in a society whose history has not allowed for the strengthening of social movements to demand their needs in all aspects of life. For this reason, there is a persistent discourse emphasizing that the state has the relevant function of educating the population so that they can redirect their conduct and attitudes:

The role of the state is not to replace popular organization, nor to create culture, but to foster it, to raise the level of consciousness, to raise the level of information. Without the state, we can't overcome this today. This country has a civil society that is still poorly organized for the demands of citizenship that we have (P1).

Finally, it is not information alone that will raise critical awareness. This can be built up with the support of EAN actions, and other educational initiatives with similar aims, which problematize issues relating to food products and related diseases in a democratic environment, allowing the population to rethink their eating practices, protect themselves from food risks and demand quality food in order to improve health and living conditions.

e) "Consent regulation"

In order to regulate market practices in the field of health, it is essential that there is a possibility, or proof, of risks that threaten the integrity of the population. The discourse of a subject linked to the international organization is emblematic and presents the technical requirements necessary to trigger a process of regulating unhealthy food products:

The relationship between the consumption of industrialized foods and these diseases (CNCDs) is clear. These foods usually have a higher amount of calories, much higher, than *fresh* food; there are some studies showing this [...] their energy density is usually higher than *fresh* food, [...] which favors the increase in excess weight in people and all the related diseases [...] (01).

However, regulation is a technical and political undertaking and, therefore, it is the discourses of the market, public authorities and Brazilian civil society, with their points of convergence and divergence, that will form the regulatory climate, explored below.

Faced with the rhetoric of the recovery of the state's regulatory power, affirmed with the institutional reform aimed at reducing bureaucratic obstacles and facilitating the development of economic activities, the reflections made by the subjects of civil society and public power flow along divergent lines. For one of them, this reform process has made the state's regulatory activity more dynamic, with the creation of regulatory agencies. For the other, there has been an inversion of the roles played by the state and the market, and a reduction in the capacity of the public authorities to interfere in the private world, leaving the latter at the mercy of economic interests:

[...] the Brazilian state has once again taken an active role, [...] it has regained its regulatory role. [...] it's just that it's not possible to believe that the market regulates and companies want it to. It's a capitalist system that is fundamentally driven by profit, and if there are no clear rules, some blockages, the consequences for the population are dramatic (S2). I really don't like this vision of the agency, this model that comes from the United States, neoliberal. [...] I have my doubts about the role of the agency as an institutional model for the state to regulate. They end up being more hostage to the market than obeying the state (P5).

It can also be seen that the entities representing the market position themselves above the interests of any fragment of society - and the way they use the values of personal indices is indicative of their supremacy: Today we export industrialized products to 114 countries [...] (M1). In the discourse of one of the market participants, the "we" alternates between two forms of expressing values: firstly, the "we" refers to the whole of Brazilian society: We happen to be a privileged country. We have everything here to feed ourselves (M1). From this perspective, he places his organization as part of society. This is his way of expressing that the measures adopted for society affect them. Today, we are a major producer (M1). There is a nationalization of "we", without distinction or conflicts.

As well as presenting itself as part of this collective organism, the national "we", the entity also presents itself as a "we", a specific body, within this national body, We are also part of this society, we produce, we employ [...] 150 years here (M1). Thus, at the same time as he insinuates that he shares common concerns as a member of the national body, he stresses in a unique way that he is the driving force behind the national body. As a differentiated part of the national body, there is a stratification that places the specific "we" (of the entity) above the national body, so that they are exempt from obeying the prescriptions of the national power: We don't need anyone to tell us what to do (M1).

This statement by the organization is often repeated, We are doing it on our own; we don't need the government; we are working with the government (M1), to reinforce the autonomy and self-sufficiency of the market in relation to government institutes, demonstrating that any interference or limitations on economic activity are unnecessary.

In fact, it is clear from the discourse that the market is an institution that can spontaneously offer its assistance to the government, and can also shape the forms of governance of power.

Even in situations where the action requires agreement between the agents involved: We made an agreement with the Ministry of Health (M3), the "we" takes on the connotation of imposition, of unilaterality, as if the initiative, willingness and decision to carry out the act fell solely on the person speaking, as one of the representatives of the market. In reality, the mobilization came from the government, due to the need to improve the nutritional quality of food products and minimize their negative impact on NCDs.

Other market participants were more permeable to interactions. In their speeches, "we" did not appear to define the specificity of the organization or the specific existence of a "we" disconnected from the collective, and there was no detachment of the entity from the collective body to assume a higher hierarchical position: I think we have various measures there (M3). We should change our habits (M2).

The food market presents itself as a sovereign and self-regulating entity, continually unleashing inventions to boost production and capital accumulation. It organizes its product innovation projects with a focus on rationalizing resources and increasing profits, and in order to make them more viable, in recent decades it has neglected some quality requirements, in this case nutritional parameters. Even after the negative effects have erupted and become collectively visible, the market continues to dissipate eating habits, impose product brands, benefit from commercial success and contribute to disease. When the risks and illnesses related to these changes in the nutritional quality of food begin to plague the population, this neoliberal idea of full independence collapses, and the state is called upon and pressured to intervene in defense of society. As far as this intervention is concerned, the discourses of market players suggest that it is sensible for the government to talk to the industries so that they gradually correct the flaws, while remaining silent about the (in our opinion, justifiable) economic impacts that could result from a legal imposition.

The experience is as follows: we think there is a way to educate, to make things happen. It's doing it together, making an effort to reduce, remove food, remove these ingredients [...]. So radicalism, regulation, closes us off and doesn't give us the flexibility that the Agreement does. The Agreement is a matter of understanding, because you can't change a formula from one moment to the next. The regulation has to be fully aware (M1).

Faced with the urgent need to reformulate the composition of food products in order to bring them closer to a healthy nutritional profile and control CNCDs, the government decided to establish formal pacts, with jointly established, flexible and long-term goals, in the form of agreements. In the view of market players, this government conduct is a demonstration of understanding between the parties, given the complexity involved in replacing the formulas of these products. For them, regulating to remedy shortcomings in a short space of time would be an inconvenient attitude on the part of the government. This is because it would imply imposing rules and establishing penalties for non-compliance. However, given that the current epidemiological panorama calls for swift intervention - and that the industries are the main culprits in the deformation of food products - the application of rules with penalties is appropriate.

With regard to this last point, one of the market participants assumes, in a subtle and thoughtful way, the industry's commitment to unhealthy products: I think there has been a huge increase in the supply of products with characteristics, or sometimes even - I'm not saying now, but until recently products with more sugar, products with excess fat [...] there was no concern about these characteristics [...] (M3).

The Ministry of Health, by taking over the functions of the regulatory body (Anvisa), was decisive in the outcome of the agreements. Anvisa was not prepared to dare to control the risks of nutrients in food products, even though these affect the health of the population. This subject completely escapes its traditional work of controlling health risks, which is concentrated on contaminants of food origin. The rigidity of the practices of the health control bodies, focused on a specific group of risks, is another element of difficulty, as it does not allow them to keep up with the health risks arising from food production technologies at the necessary speed. This would require liaison with stakeholders and adjustments to regulations and procedures in order to provide effective responses to protect society in a timely manner. This institutional distancing from emerging health risks therefore prevents the regulatory body from acting to safeguard the health of the population from the harms of unhealthy food products.

Regulation and regulation are referred to as synonyms in the speech of certain subjects: He has to oblige [...]. He has to regulate (S3). When I say regulate, I mean that it has to be standardized, that there have to be clear rules and even sanctions (S2). As already defined in this paper, **regulation** involves a list of legal and compulsory technical and administrative control measures that the institution has in place to protect the health of the population from health risks arising from the food production system. And in the case of health, **regulation** is understood as the development of a set of legal and mandatory provisions that the public administration imposes on third parties to preserve the health of the population, including sanctions.

The consensus-building between the government and the market entities, formalized in the Public-Private Partnership Agreement in the field of health, can reflect balanced concessions or losses for one of the parties. The government's choice not to regulate, or rather, to dispense with the use of this prerogative in favor of the Partnership Agreement, signals a retreat by the government in favor of the market, since, alternatively, a regulation could have been drawn up, through a participatory, dialogical and democratic construction process between all the interested parties, with a negotiated legal deadline. This is the impression given by one of the individuals from civil society: I think there's this view today - public-private partnership - that actually, [...] I perceive there's a risk [...] of privatization, of granting power, as if the market could regulate (S2).

The opinions expressed by market participants on the measures (agreement and regulation) are wide-ranging. When making parallel comparisons, there is a clear opposition in the qualifications attributed to each of them. The former is seen as a symbol of understanding, dialogue, the common good, consensus, rationality and education; in short, the protector of the market. Regulation, on the other hand, represents radicalism, control, authoritarianism, inefficiency and inflexibility. It is striking how a regulatory practice that has been in place for decades, and which has the function of regulating the market to protect the collective interests of health, and to make competition between companies fair, becomes an instrument of controversy, in the view of those involved in the market. This occurs even in the face of the market's proven inability to manage itself in order to offer quality products to the population: [...] I get a little shivery when someone starts talking about industrialized foods having to be regulated, I'm against these controls. We are fully aware that the industries based here are fully aware of what control is (M1).

Also noteworthy is the use of the pronoun "we", which takes on a value that does not encompass the industrial world, nor the Brazilian people, but is limited to the group that the subject represents.

The discourse of this same subject, in continuation, emphasizes that, in an effort to update production capacity, companies invest in technologies that value commercial aspects and quality control of the risk parameters that they believe affect the performance of their economic activity:

[...] the technology, with the modernism to present it to the consumer in a more appropriate way, [...] so that it can be consumed healthily and with a guarantee that it won't harm them. [...] they have absolutely complete laboratories, often superior to the laboratories of government control agents. Therefore, the quality response they give is much more accurate, much more precise than any laboratory anywhere, at any university (M1).

However, it has to be considered that companies choose and monitor the analytical, health and other parameters that could jeopardize the trade in their products. It is clear that nutritional parameters are excluded from the list of their controls, because they are not yet recognized as a health risk, either by the companies themselves or by the government. At the moment, these parameters are still dispensable from the market's point of view.

Before having the function of modernizing products, these technologies must necessarily result in advantages and profits, even if, paradoxically, they can also cause unforeseen effects that result in adversities and health risks. And, in general, if these negative effects don't affect the profitability of capital, they are only recognized by the market when they are elucidated in research carried out by public research centers. And even then, the results of these studies always tend to be minimized or exposed to controversy when they require a change in the production model - in the case of food products with an unhealthy profile. The presence of the neologism "healthiness" in this statement subtly shifts the focus from the product to the gesture of consuming, in other words, to the conditions of how consumption is carried out, in order to remove any controversy surrounding the product.

The controversy over the control of chronic health effects caused by unhealthy food products is pertinent to the following comment. Threats of this nature - extensive, long-lasting, imperceptible to the layperson in the early stages, with serious consequences and a high cost to society - only the state is capable of transforming them into a social issue, given its responsibility, by shaping them into a policy of market regulation in the field of health:

Nobody can expect the market to be spontaneously compatible with social rights, especially health rights, because it is geared towards profit. So it always needs to be regulated, socially controlled and with the state being its biggest component (P5).

The competitiveness that governs the food market reflects, to a certain extent, the lack of cohesion and the existence of a system of stratification between companies. It is a hierarchy of power between industrial corporations, which makes smaller industries, or those linked to less politically significant entities, almost obliged to follow the conduct or adopt the procedures of first-rate industries in order to remain in the market:

We are the vast majority - [...] the top two hundred companies in the country in terms of production. If we make the product lower, the others will have to keep up or they'll lose the market. Our companies are already ahead and to set an example we offered this - let's work together in this business, because you won't be able to do it alone (M1).

Therefore, the profile of entities chosen by the government to undertake initiatives to promote the adaptation of food products included industries with high economic power and products with wide national and international circulation. Therefore, a strategic segment for the Agreement.

With the current characteristics in the composition of food products, it cannot be said that these entities in the production sector are exemplary in terms of their ethical and social commitments. It can only be said that they set a standard of consumption of unhealthy products for society. However, due to their economic presence in the market, when they decide to reduce the content of those nutrients that are considered harmful to health, other industries may be forced to apply this measure to their products, due to competition.

As explained above, the debate that preceded the construction of the government's Agreement with the entities was restricted to the productive sector, and the subjects of organized civil society criticize this initiative: [...] society was not summoned and neither was academia [...]. It was the Ministry of Health and the industries who took part in this agreement, with the support of Anvisa (S1). However, for the government: Politics is about dialog, because this is what democracy is all about. This doesn't mean alignment. It means dialog, the search for convergent agendas and dialog with the food industry (P2). These arguments give rise to a clear confrontation between the "exercise of democracy" and the "extension of representation". Extending democratic practice in public spaces necessarily requires the participation of all stakeholders in the deliberations of a collective body (BOBBIO, 2005). In this case, the absence of civil society in this institutional dialog compromises both the legitimacy of the deliberations adopted and demonstrates a step backwards in participatory management.

One of the individuals linked to civil society comments: "These agreements are necessary, but they are insufficient and timid in terms of their goals. Firstly, they are Agreements that only concern sodium; while we already know that the problem is not limited to sodium [...] they are weak goals that require little or no effort from industry (S1).

As already discussed in this study, the key nutrients of health interest to be reduced in food products are fats, sugars and salt; however, the negotiation was limited to the sodium (salt) content, leaving the other nutrients to be discussed *a posteriori*, in a new round of negotiations. This demonstrates the political difficulties of revising nutrients en bloc.

This initiative - to proceed with Agreements - breaks with Brazil's institutional tradition in the field of food regulation, which did not include, in its practical provisions, monitoring the results of voluntary Agreements formalized with the industries[36] . The law and its complementary regulations, instruments of a compulsory nature and with provision for sanctions, have always been used in the regular practice of the sanitary control body to discipline the behavior of food industries. This change in intervention strategy was beneficial for the industries in two ways: a) it allowed them to extend the time for their products to comply; and, b) it avoided subjecting them to penalties for non-compliance with the Agreement. This is how the voices of civil society put it: [...] government activity today is more about relaxing than tightening regulations (S1). Now it doesn't go through the Agreement, [...] it has to go through the requirement. It's an appropriate measure, but it's very tenuous. [...] because what's at stake is the health of the population (S3).

The explanation for this attitude is purely political, because the seriousness of the Brazilian morbidity and mortality pattern and its interrelationship with food products, proven by scientific studies and supranational organizations, justifies the implementation of an incisive measure by the government. However, the lack of internal political will to face up to the pressures of the industries, which are opposed to this type of measure, and the absence of an effective counterpoint from society, has led the government to back down and opt for slowly achieving the desired objectives for food products.

If it were a compulsory nationwide rule on food control, the effect would cover all industries, forcing them to reduce the levels of unhealthy nutrients within a specified period. As a result, any industry, regardless of its will, would be obliged to reduce the levels of these nutrients or face legal sanctions. Therefore, this rule would supersede the

36 The state health surveillance agencies and the central public health laboratories - LACEN - take part in monitoring the foods involved in the agreement, in order to verify compliance with the established targets.

scope of the Agreement's administrative act, which is restricted only to those industries linked to the entities that have ratified the document in question. However, the government's choice was to involve a few entities representing the food production sector, but constituting a relevant conglomerate of industries, both in economic terms and in terms of the market penetration of their products. Thus, when asked about the Agreement, one of the civil society members replied: What is the only value of these Agreements today, from a symbolic point of view, I would say? [...] is to bring this issue to public attention, but effectively in terms of health. The issue of hate has really reached everyone's ears. So everyone is more or less sensitized to it (S1).

Global companies, through their interlocutors and with the intention of preserving their interests, maintain an active channel of international articulation with the units of their food industry networks. Among its tasks are to inform its member organizations of the criticism, pressure and mobilization at the international level by countries, civil society organizations and international bodies in relation to food products, and to advise them on how best to defend themselves in these situations. The movement to change the nutritional profile of food products is not a local initiative, but an international trend, backed by the WHO and FAO, which are paying attention to NCDs. This has already aroused the attention of the market's corporate entities, compelling them to communicate to their members about the need to rethink their formulas, in order to anticipate possible incisive action by governments in this field:

[...] the multinationals brought this idea, because when they make an application at a certain time, they extend it to the rest of the world. So they were told that, at a certain point, they had to start thinking about it [...]. The formulas had already been studied there, to see what the alternatives were; what the substitute was, etc. So we started long before the government woke up to the problem (M1).

It can be seen that the liaison between national and international companies only resulted in the exchange of information. No action was taken until the government came forward. Ethical concerns about certain risks of food products and their involvement with NCDs are outside the scope of interest of the global market. To deal with this issue, the industries act only under political pressure.

The interference of the decisions of intergovernmental food regulation bodies in the internal functioning of the country is evident, both on the part of the public authorities and the market. In public discourse, the reference denotes a mixture of dependence and impotence, implying a partial loss of national sovereignty to make its own rules, even in the face of justifications considered relevant to health:

The process of agreeing a regulatory measure involves, especially in the area of food, an international agreement, because it's Mercosur [...]. The progress of the regulatory agenda (nutritional components) will depend, firstly, on international tension, as seen in other agendas, and on the building of a chain of support for the MoH [...] and obviously concerted action, support from society [...] (P4).

Despite the external commitments, in the final section of this speech, it becomes clear that the government depends on the power of society, which is relevant and strategic in defining the direction of decisions, including dealing with controversial issues such as the regulation of nutritional components in food products, which could lead it to move forward in its proposals, beyond what has been agreed in the international pacts.

On the market side, the relationship established with supranational and intragovernmental bodies is seen as a means of expressing their intentions and exerting their influence on the course of decisions, despite reporting apparently limited action:

[...] we also end up participating in the discussion within Brazil and then indirectly even sometimes as an observer at *Codex* [...]. For positioning, not voting or vetoing, but positioning before *Codex.* And in Mercosur, we end up taking part in the different committees through Anvisa (M3).

When convenient, these instances are reported and recognized as having a higher *status* than the state; for example, when a market participant mentions the elasticity of the deadline for adapting food product formulas in terms of sodium content: In our formulas we will reach 2020 as recommended by the World Organization [...] (M1).

Within the group of public authorities and civil society, there is no uniformity of positions on the subject of the agreement. There were three clearly defined positions on the formalized agreements between the government and the industries, namely: a) favorable, and it is up to the government to overcome differences of interest with the industries, [...] the government needs to be a partner with our industries (P4); It's a governance measure combined with the industrial segment (P3); b) conditional on preserving the supremacy of the public interest and other prerogatives inherent to the state, I don't see any problems in signing agreements, as long as they don't have counterparts that hurt the state (P1); and c) against, because the content negotiated is relevant to public health, as well as being feasible to implement in legal form, I am totally in favor of legislating what can be legislated without hindrance and for the good of the population. I am in favor of regulation, unless a deadline is set for compliance with the rules (P5).

The Agreement shows the clear intention of the Ministry of Health and Anvisa, as government bodies, to choose an intervention strategy that would produce the least political wear and tear for the government and the least economic impact for the market: first, a rule should have been made; since that wasn't possible, an Agreement was made, because there was an interest in not harming the national industry (P6). The Agreement, then, was designed to ease the conflicts, avoid turbulence in the economic field, avoid direct clashes with organized civil society and, finally, gradually adjust the quality of food products, despite the epidemiological situation they cause.

The discourse of the market is presented as the savior of the economy and of the state itself, due to its contribution to employment, its importance in the balance of trade and the taxes it transfers and which guarantee the functioning of the state machine: [...] except that we produce, we employ, we pay taxes, we export, we've been there for 150 years (M1). This speech demonstrates both economic and political strength, and implicitly intimidates the government, compelling it to back down from making more consistent political arrangements, in order to save itself from possible threats and retaliation.

In addition, the Public-Private Partnership in question alters the government's standardized routine and changes the way food control is done, which could have worrying consequences, such as: a) the resulting significant ideological effect, which covers up conflicts and leads to a false neutralization of the differences between government and private purposes, creating the false illusion in society of substantial advances in the public interest; b) the weakening of the legal and legitimate nature of the authority of the public authorities to impose obligations on the private sector, a function now described by the market as authoritarianism; and c) the creation of precedents for the market to press for an interactive relationship based on understanding and partnership, rather than compulsory rules, when confronting and defending issues of public interest.

In this sense, one of the discourses of the subjects of public power is illustrative in praising this flexibility in the actions of public power in relation to the market:

[...] it's no longer possible to do the surveillance of arriving, fining, seizing, that we used to do when health surveillance was created. Today, modern health surveillance works with *stakeholders*, with partnerships and I think this is a contemporary movement. It's about bringing the industry into responsibility, showing it the importance and voluntariness, and getting it to make this change; but this has a deadline (P4).

Administrative acts, which are recognized as legal and necessary to be applied in situations of health risks for the benefit of the public, become a derogatory, outdated and inappropriate image in the contemporary context, for those who are guided by the motto "the market can do anything". It should be noted that this position is not hegemonic within the public power group, according to excerpts from the speeches mentioned above and the following speech: I don't think Anvisa can shirk this responsibility, because it has to regulate and it can't be left in the wake of the market. These are the difficulties of stronger legislation in order to act (P5). The difference between this discourse and the previous one lies in the interpretation that public-private interaction and dispensing with the use of legislation is a timid and subservient behavior on the part of the public authorities towards the market. It is therefore incompatible with social relevance and inappropriate for dealing with the affairs of the community.

Referring to Bourdieu's (2009) concept, it can be seen that food regulation fits in perfectly as a field of symbolic production, constituting a space of social power relations, where truths clash and interests conflict. The social effects are shaped by consensus or divergence, originating in the behavior and intentions of the agents involved, and culminating in impositions that are defined and redefined along the continuous path of the political struggle. At the moment the Agreement prevails, tomorrow the Regulation may be in force.

In order to give a synthetic overview of the matrix statements, postulates and discursive realizations that have been addressed, Table 4 is presented below.

TABLE 4: Summary of matrix statements on food risks and regulation.

MATRIX STATEMENTS	POSTULATES	SPEECH PERFORMANCES	INTERPRETATIONS/ COMMENTS
Essence of the food	Food is essentially life. Food's identity is untouchable, and interference is incapable of stripping it of its mythical purity. Balanced food consumption translates into health and life.	• *[...] Food is one of the fundamental things in human life (MI).* • *Food influences health in many ways [...] (P4).* • *This consumerist logic that leads to obesity [...] (PI).* • *The sweetening of*	Although food is mythologized as a source of energy and life for humanity, and industrial processing is used to restore its vital properties and increase its shelf life, in recent times the essential character of food has been distorted, displacing

		these foods is undoubtedly very much linked to the damage done to health today - the amount of sugar, salt (P5).	it from nutrition. The change in the composition of food and the marketing gimmicks used to stimulate consumption, combined with urban lifestyles, have had harmful effects on people's health.

TABLE 4: Summary of matrix statements on food risks and regulation. [Continued]

MATRIX STATEMENTS	POSTULATES	DISCURSIVE Performances	INTERPRETATIONS/ COMMENTS
Irreversibility of the industrialized product	It discusses the economic logic of food production (exclusively for profit and/or health benefits) and the food product, the result of a technological process, comparing it with the authenticity (real or imagined) of food extracted from nature.	•*Industrialized food is a necessity [...] (M2).* •*Industrialized foods are interwoven into modern life [...] (P6).* •*The obesity pandemic is linked to the market. [...] there are foods that are addictive - soft drinks are addictive, sugar is addictive (PI).* •*The industry [...] is putting better nutritional products on the market. Now it depends on the social class that can access it (M2).* •*[...] There's no point in reducing our product. It won't make our product fat, it will make the rest fat, with everything (Ml).* •*Fat and sugar bring flavor to food. So, if you want to captivate an audience so that they eat that food, the side of the person who is designing the food will say: load up on sai; load up on sugar and load up on fat (SI).*	The food product meets the expectations of urbanites due to its versatility, being practical, affordable and having disposable packaging. It also boosts the consumer economy through constant innovation and product substitution. he technology used in food production has a contradictory character, because while it provides certain quality requirements for the product, it also has devastating negative impacts: it disrupts food culture, creates physical dependency and generates different types of illness. However, it should be noted that the quality of the product acts as a social marker and forms two groups: those considered to have a better nutritional profile and are more expensive, and those that are less healthy, pose a greater risk to health and cost less, which are

			consumed by the poorest sections of the population. At this point, some market players are more inclined to agree with the need to reformulate products to meet nutritional and health requirements.

TABLE 4: Summary of matrix statements on food risks and regulation (Continued)

MATRIX STATEMENTS	POSTULATES	SPEECH PERFORMANCES	INTERPRETATIONS/ COMMENTS
Consumer Implication	The individual, under the neoliberal prism, is autonomous in making his or her food choices and is the bearer of knowledge and experiences that enable him or her to take responsibility for protecting themselves from the risks that affect their own health.	• *[...] the increase in sedentary lifestyles [...] people are becoming more and more complacent [...] they don't exercise or do less physical activity. It's not just about food (M2).* • *[...] it is the consumer himself who is to blame for overeating and its consequences - it is the human being who, in greed, greed, gluttony, overdoes what he does or doesn't prepare himself properly who is to blame. (Ml).* • *(...) but the population has been greatly encouraged and has become aware, although not to the extent that is desirable; (...) of the importance of food in a person's life (S3).* • *There is a reasonable sample who have more access to information and are more sensitive, but they don't always act in practice (P5).*	The individual, who is part of contemporary society governed by the neoliberal spirit, is indoctrinated to create self-protection mechanisms against risks, such as practicing self-care, aiming for the integrity of their health and keeping their body regulated. Otherwise, they may deviate from this established order. In the case of food risks, the consumer can take two positions: guilty or victim. From the point of view of the market, they are guilty of overeating, not paying attention to product labeling and living a sedentary lifestyle; from the point of view of the public authorities and civil society, they tend to be victims for submitting to market pressures and for lacking adequate information about food.

TABLE 4: Summary of matrix statements on food risks and regulation. [Continued]

MATRIX STATEMENTS	POSTULATES	SPEECH PERFORMANCES	INTERPRETAMES/ COMMENTS

Consumer to trans (form)	The consumer's capacity for self-defense lies in the information transmitted, which acts as an engine for transforming their awareness and conduct.	• *The government is making the biggest mistake in history, looking only at the industrialized and not focusing on the rest and we are not the whole; we are a part. The government has to educate (MI).* • *The role of the state is not to replace popular organization, [...] but to encourage it, to raise the level of consciousness, to raise the level of information (Pl).* • *[...] it is important that this issue of food is not concentrated in the space of organized civil society alone, citizens need to take on this reflection, because I don't think we have the strength to move this agenda (P2).*	Education is presented as the only means capable of transforming the behavior of individuals and the population in relation to the practice of food consumption, in order to control the risks arising from it. Information must be used to empower the population, but without relieving the state of its duty to curb the excesses committed by the market, which has repercussions on social life. It should also be pointed out that, given the historical weakness of social movements and their distance from food issues, the state is responsible for disseminating information so that the population raises its awareness and acquires autonomy to manage its food consumption.

TABLE 4: Summary of matrix statements on food risks and regulation (Continued)

MATRIX STATEMENTS	**POSTULATES**	**SPEECH PERFORMANCES**	**INTERPRETATIONS/ COMMENTS**
"Consented regulation"	The achievement of a healthy product is not limited exclusively to legal provisions, but involves regulatory governance, agreed between the interested parties, reconciling the interests of the market and society.	- *The experience is as follows: we think there is a way to educate, to make things happen. Doing things together, making an effort to reduce, remove food, remove these ingredients [...]. So it's radicalism, a regulation that closes off and doesn't give the flexibility that the Agreement does. The Agreement is a thing of understanding, you can't change a formula from one moment to the next. The regulation has to be fully*	The formal pacts established by the government with the industries to reformulate the nutritional profile of food products is the subject of controversy in the interests of the market, public authorities and civil society. When discussing the agreement and the regulations, the market

		aware (MI). • *These agreements are necessary, but insufficient and timid in terms of their* goals. *[...] they are weak goals that require no or very little effort from industry (SI).* • *I think Anvisa can't shirk this responsibility, the park has to standardize and can't be left in the wake of the market. There are difficulties in getting stronger legislation to act (P5).* • *I think there's this vision today of a Private-Private Partnership - which, in fact, [...] I perceive has a risk [...] of privatization, of granting power, if only the market could regulate (S2).*	believes that the former symbolizes a manifestation of understanding and accessibility, while the latter represents radicalism and authoritarianism on the part of the government. Public authorities and civil society express different points of view on the issue: One side admits the need for the Agreement but affirms the fragility of the targets and considers that the government has backed down in the face of industry's demands, given the seriousness of the epidemiological situation; for another, the fact that the regulator has refrained from adopting regulations with a provision for sanctions means that it is placing itself in a position of subservience to the market, which reveals the weakness of the body responsible for promoting the well-being of the whole community.

6.2 "Food" and "Nutrition": generation and variations in discursive positions

By exploring the matrix statements, two elementary semantic terms stood out in the construction of the discourses, ***food*** and ***nutrition,*** from which arises a range of meanings with distinct possibilities of variation, which can be exposed using the topology of the semiotic square, first developed by Greimas (1970), to think about the programming and circulation of the objects of discourse and their values.

The application of the Semiotic Square model in this thesis is merely illustrative, with the aim of raising the possibility of exploring the semantic terms of Nutrition through this model. However, it should be emphasized that this is not intended to exhaust the discussion on its applicability and validation in the field of Nutrition.

Considering that meaning is something that is constructed, the semiotic square is based on the assumption that all discourse follows a model of competence that puts into play a relationship between four terms, conceived as the foundation of its significant structure. This square refers to the idea that any narrative is based on a dual relationship between the notion and its semantic opposite (food *versus* nutrition), each of these poles implying its contradictory (non-food and non-nutrition), as shown in Figure 1.

In this way, all discourse emanates from the realization of a constant and discontinuous path, from one position to another, on these two axes (the axis of contradiction implying that of sub-contradiction). In its development, this path generates its meanings, according to the narrative and figurative program projected by the fundamental quaternary relationship, and varying according to the universe of action of its enunciator. In short, the square represents, in a syntactic way, how the production of meaning, in its multiple variations, is circumscribed within a given semantic field. According to Barros (2005), this visual representation shows, on the one hand, how an elementary structure intricate in a network of relationships is reduced to a single relationship and, on the other, how the purity of difference does not exist and escapes the dynamics of the social world.

In this sense, Figure 1 shows the different possible meanings that circulate in this semantic field:

- ***The food/nutrition axis:*** This ***is*** a discourse in which the whole person is seen, endowed with freedom and autonomy to organize their way of life. A being who is also a citizen, who enjoys a set of rights that enable them to have decent conditions to maintain their life and, therefore, the integrity of their health. In this way, they are aware and qualified to consume in a balanced way and benefit from food products that meet their nutritional needs, their food culture and also provide them with pleasure. As an agent of a democratic process, their presence in the collective is geared towards defending and fighting for collective demands, leaving the others as subordinate: We really value the achievement we had of including in the Constitution - the right to adequate and healthy food as part of article 60, which talks about social rights (S2). It is from this perspective that a food and nutrition security policy is designed, integrating the different facets of the food production system and enabling the realization of everyone's right to regular access to food, in terms of quantity and quality, compatible with cultural values and production linked to an economically, socially and environmentally sustainable policy.

Figure 1: Food & nutrition semiotic square.

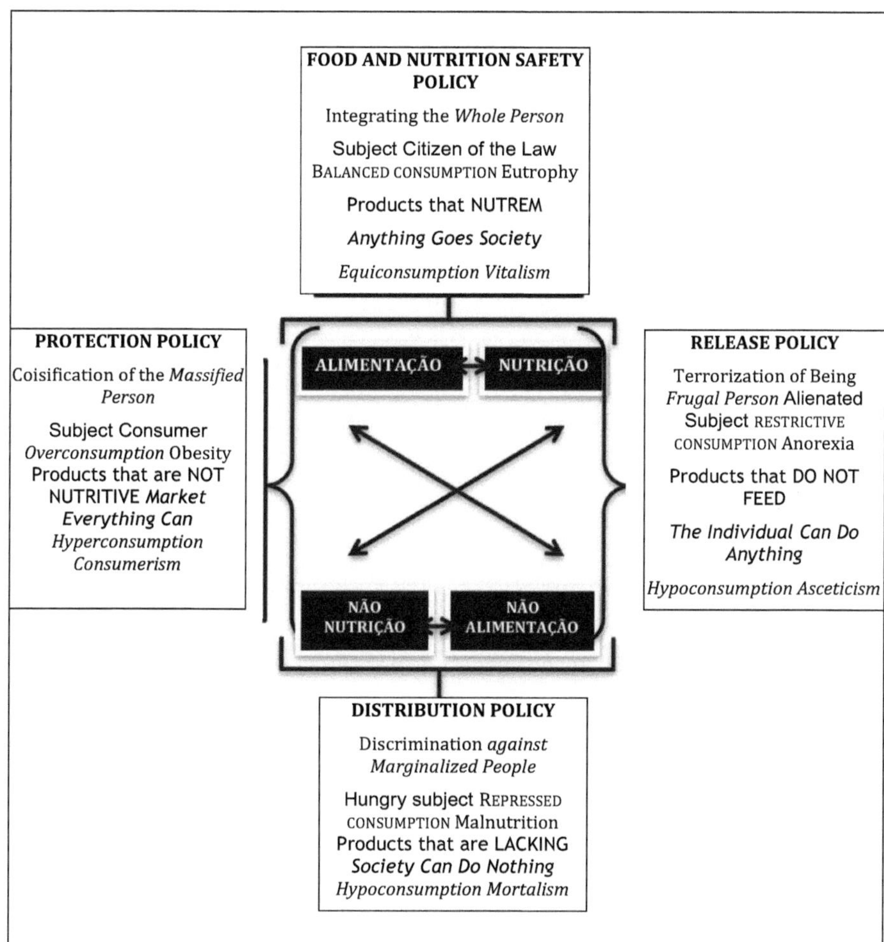

The non-nutrition/non-feeding axis: This is the opposite axis, in which the discourse is inverted in its content. The being is reduced to a sub-category of the human race, deprived of the essential means to enable the fullness of life, and only natural instinct makes it resist and survive in the face of society's contempt. The unlimited consumption of food doesn't satisfy hunger and degrades health, producing deficiencies and other illnesses, which only help to speed up the end of the individual's or collective existence: [...] it's not by starving, it's not with a diet that doesn't meet that person's needs, but in a process of changing habits (S3). According to Valente (2003), with their human right to adequate food denied, excluded from citizenship and not worthy of equal *status* in a stratified and segregated society, these quasi-citizens depend on a distributive and socially just public policy, aimed at guaranteeing everyone access to food in qualitative and quantitative terms, in order to satisfy their nutritional needs, enable stable health, increase life expectancy and, above all, recognize them as citizens with rights.

***The nutrition/non-nutrition axis*:** The discourse that derives from this points to the massacre of the human being as it is guided by the values of body aesthetics that make up the dominant ideology, which also defines the criteria for social and personal acceptance and, concomitantly, guides dietary practices (CONTRERAS & GRACIA, 2011). The individual then has to "voluntarily" deprive themselves of food consumption, allowing themselves to obtain only the minimum fuel necessary for life. If they think that too much food has been consumed, they quickly expel it, keeping themselves under "rigid control". The rejection of food doesn't happen in isolation; it goes hand in hand with the rejection of pleasure, both of which compromise health. This situation ends up leading to a process of lack of interest in life. The individual, a free and autonomous being, is predisposed to submit to the social pressures that dictate the ideal body profile and, when faced with failures, sees them as a matter of moral failure. As this individual behavior multiplies, it becomes a social issue. The movement required is aimed at freeing citizens from this ideological oppression, rethinking and repressing the means and strategies used, especially by the media, to disseminate these deformed values of body aesthetics.

- ***The food/non-nutrition axis:*** The discourse begins by reducing the subject to an object. According to Bauman (2008), in today's society, consumption is seen as the vocation of every individual, in other words, as a universal human right and duty. Thus, the subject is captured by the market and becomes a victim of inducement to compulsively buy goods, in this case, food products, to the point of losing their self-control and compromising their own health: We need to free the human being inside each consumer, so that the human being is not diminished and the condition of the consumer is aggravated, so that as much information as possible is available about the food that is provided in public spaces (P5).

In the field of food, consumerism takes the form of a constantly diversified and socially differentiated range of products, which are constantly being renewed and publicized in order to arouse consumers' interests and desires: This consumerist logic leads to obesity, not just of the body, but obesity of the mind, of the senses. Consumerism is an expression of today's society and it has a lot to do with drug addiction, not least because it means the search for immediate, flashy pleasure (P1).

The market is not democratized, but stratified, and begins to supply products for the enjoyment of the poorest consumer groups. These are food products with a differentiated profile that carry certain attributes such as: inferior nutritional quality, low price, high taste power and symbolic expression of social *status*:

The industry [...] is putting more nutritious products on the market. Now it depends on the social class that can afford it. The more people can afford it, the more they will look for this type of product. So, if you had a greater volume of production, you could reduce it, but it's already more expensive (M1).

Food products that satisfy hunger but, on the other hand, don't nourish and create food insecurity problems for consumers. To curb the market's excesses, protective measures are needed - such as those that regulate the nutritional quality of food and its advertising and promote healthy eating - to re-establish health-promoting food practices: Nobody can expect the market to be spontaneously compatible with social rights, especially health rights, because it is geared towards profit. So it must always be regulated, socially controlled and with the state being its biggest component (P5). In order to be a conscious consumer, the individual needs to acquire the *status of* a citizen, i.e. one who is free and autonomous to make choices and reflective before making decisions.

As shown in the Semiotic Square (Figure 1), the set of positions taken by the interviewees' speeches (concentrated between the food/nutrition dichotomy and the non-food/non-nutrition subcontradiction) produces different meanings, according to the thematic role that the enunciators adopt and refer to the other, as subjects and social actors. Although the visual representation of the terms food/nutrition has made it possible to shape the different types of discourse studied, the controversial positions were essentially located on the axes ***food/non-nutrition*** (which discusses the quality of industrialized food) and ***food/nutrition*** (which questions the alternatives for achieving a balance of food and nutrition for all). Although the themes of the other two axes (***non-food/non-nutrition*** and ***nutrition/non-food***) are not present in the corpus analyzed, they refer to discursive potentialities that may or may not appear according to the contexts and protagonists of the enunciation, in the form of delineations of a counter-discourse whose effects have already been overcome (extreme food poverty and the hungry subject, in the case of the ***non-nutrition/non-food*** axis); or which are not significant enough to justify systematic action by the public authorities (eating disorders, in the case of the ***nutrition/non-food*** axis).

The diagram represents an incipient approach to narrative theory and was drawn up with the intention of briefly demonstrating, in a clear and quick way - but also highlighting the complex interdependence of the representations at play - the evidence identified of conjunctions and disjunctions of reflections and actions between the discourses of the different subjects surveyed and linked to each of these *loci* of action - the market, public authorities or civil society.

In view of the above, this schematization, as well as the interpretations and comments derived from it, aim to delimit precisely, but without exhausting, the dialectic of the intersections between each one, the significant set formed by the discourses. From our perspective, it also aims to trace how the logics of action work, in an attempt to answer the question of which representations (imaginary and pragmatic), concordances, displacements, oppositions and how the subjects view the generic and specific interconnection of the processes of food and nutrition, and the possible transformations, considering the attractive forces of the market, political power and society.

6.3 Regulating food risks: ideologies, interests and power

Thompson's concept of ideology (THOMPSON, 2000), as mentioned at the beginning of this paper, refers to the different ways in which the FS and the meaning they mobilize construct social reality, and serve to **establish** and **sustain** power relations. These are two actions centered on "meaning", with specific but interdependent purposes, whose joint effect guides the process of understanding and realizing ideology. The first shows how meaning, as an active and continuous creation, establishes relations of domination between groups and people; and the second reveals how meaning acts to maintain and reproduce relations of domination, through a dynamic pathway of production and reception of FS.

Understanding the KS as ideological depends on this interactive relationship of meaning and power, which is inseparable from the socially structured context in which it is operationalized. With regard to this contextual aspect, the author starts from the assumption that the distribution of and access to the various types of resources is not uniform for people *and* groups. It is systematic differentiations that allow people and groups, by virtue of their position in the social context and the (intellectual and economic) qualifications they have incorporated, to appropriate different quantities of resources and different degrees of access to them.

He also clarifies that these resources are, in fact, degrees of power, understood as the capacity that certain people have, socially or institutionally, to transform the reality of social facts: to influence decisions, achieve their objectives and realize their interests. He also points out that "power" necessarily implies systematically asymmetrical relationships. It is particular groups that, in comparison to others, have a different *amount of* power, in a permanent and relevant way, regardless of the situation in question.

The grouped discourses of the market, the government and civil society regarding the regulation of the nutritional components of food products in order to interfere with the profile of NCDs are versions of an event in social reality, constructed collectively, with styles, plots and arguments specific to each of these representations. Ideology is the essential constituent of these discourses, responsible for mobilizing meanings and revealing how they intersect with relations of domination, shaping and distinguishing discourses, as well as making conflicts and inequalities of interest explicit.

The ideology of the discourses on food regulation flows in a similar way to a board game with three strategic pieces that, as they move, reveal the plot of power, which will be summarized below. For the **market**, what interests it is the accumulation of capital. It wants to take advantage of technological advances to improve and expand the production and marketing of food products, in order to continually unsettle consumers with its diversified products. To do this, it uses its economic and political power to remove any obstacles that threaten the success of this venture. The advent of economic globalization has only strengthened this position. Companies have taken on a new reconfiguration on the world stage, forming corporations and becoming protagonists of the world's economic map. These transnational corporations are detached from a specific geographic space and are able to distribute their products across the globe, influence the decisions of public authorities, maintain and make their business viable, including making competition between their peers fair. They are also beginning to interfere in the supranational and local institutions that regulate the food trade, exerting a marked influence on the decisions made in these instances. Faced with the need to boost profits, these corporations reconfigure the nutritional profile of food products in a uniform way, with cheap, low-nutrient and low-cost ingredients; they then adopt a variety of strategies to homogenize the pattern of consumption and dissolve the kaleidoscope of cultural values and eating practices present in societies. For the market, the "idiosyncrasies" of food products come from the consumer, who is inactive and consumes too much. The result of this "global economic progress" is, in addition to exorbitant private profit, health risks (NCDs), which are continually expanding across the planet.

Public authorities are increasingly called upon to intervene and discipline the market in the face of food risks that are becoming more complex with sophisticated technologies. But before acting, it is obliged to consider the international and regional pacts - Mercosur - which limit the freedom and autonomy of its own action, as well as assessing its internal capacity and the repercussions of a potential intervention. The weakened structure of public power reveals the political difficulty of countering market interests. The solution to circumvent the externalities of the food market, reflected in the field of health, is mitigated by the use of unusual and weak instruments (Agreements) compared to compulsory and punitive rules, to reduce the harmful nutritional components present in these products. This Agreement, signed between the government and industrial entities, not only represents a deviation from the institutionalized routine, but was drawn up in the midst of compromised governance, without the presence of organized civil society. The powerful pressure of the market, combined with the political fragility of the government, means that the former determines that social interests should be negotiated gradually, through agreements that imply minimal readjustments to the market.

Thus, faced with an unequal balance of power between the entities, the Agreement was the option chosen by the government to manage the divergent interests between the market and the community. However, the impasse between guaranteeing health or interfering with the accelerated pace of capital accumulation has not yet been overcome.

Organized civil society, although aware of the risks of food and the need for regulation, recognizes the incipient mobilization of the collective and the importance of sensitizing social groups to include this issue on their agendas. They have limited power to confront the interests of the market and achieve immediate success. However, society's lack of active and systematic participation in decision-making processes to contain food risks compromises both the way it voices its health interests and its ability to influence the actions of public authorities in order to value collective demands. In this way, the aspiration to effectively prevent diseases, which in part derive from the unhealthy conduct of the market, is delayed, as is the guarantee of the full right to health.

Considering these three sets of speeches that address the validity of public regulation as a strategy to control the risks of the nutritional composition of food products, establishing its extent and limitations, it is also possible to highlight the dominant feature of each group's discourse and then classify it according to Thompson's (2000) typology on the *modus operandi* of ideology.

The first series of speeches, coming from the market group, speaks the language of economic interests, in which the intrinsic quality of food, together with the efficiency of the free functioning of the market, ensure progress in production, making it possible for all sections of society to have access to food products, which requires limited intervention by public authorities. Here, ideology operates through ***legitimization***, using the strategy of ***universalization***, in which the interests of one group are presented as being at the service of the collective.

The second series, represented by the public authorities, speaks the language of the institutional duty to regulate food, in favor of maintaining and improving the market, through laws or agreements, so that the market can satisfy everyone's needs, according to society's wishes. In this case, ideology is ***legitimized*** through the strategy of ***rationalization***, which uses a logical sequence of reasoning, with an appeal to legality, to defend or justify a practice or procedure.

The third tier, which brings together the civil society group, speaks the language of citizens' rights; the individual is the bearer of broad and extensive rights, such as the right to health, won in a democratic society. These rights define the limits of the market and also those of the state, which must not be exceeded by the actions of these two actors. The ideology's mode of operation is that of ***unification,*** through the strategy of ***standardization***, in which emphasis is placed on the importance of improving the nutritional quality of food products for everyone's health. This distinction is based on shared and acceptable technical-political foundations, which serve to create a collective unity between groups of citizens, regardless of the different contexts in which they consume food.

Despite the specific ideological markers of each group of subjects, what stands out is a world governed by neoliberal ideology, where the market and society follow their courses within normality; the one who stands out is the individual, who is not able to have an effective and healthy relationship with their diet, in other words, they consume too many food products and adopt a sedentary lifestyle, contrary to the expectations that the market and public power have of them. This doctrine is based on linear thinking, reduced to the economic dimension, anchored in the market, which is totally incompatible with a vision of a solidary and just society. But, for now, it is still a hegemonic vision.

CONCLUSION

Contemporary society in general, when inserted into a context of economic and cultural globalization, loses the reference between the local and the global when it comes to emerging food risks. The institutions representing the state, for their part, are shedding some of their local sovereignty, opting to act in an agreed manner with the supranational actors that regulate world food trade, such as the WHO, FAO and WTO. Meanwhile, corporations and transnational conglomerates make use of technical and intellectual resources to develop new products, expand markets and boost global capital. These are the global players, the ones who devise different types of cartographies of the world, for economic and political purposes, to influence government decisions at national, regional and international level. It is under this set of influences that market regulation by national government takes place.

Based on these considerations, regulating emerging food risks is a challenging task for national governments. The prescriptions of the competent international organizations, encouraging and calling on states to intervene in food products with high levels of saturated fats, sugars and salt, are insufficient. It should be noted that the high prevalence of obesity and other CNCDs, and the pressure from transnational industries uninterested in modifying these products, which are important sources of profit, create an environment of conflicts and tensions in order to regulate food. Regulation aimed at preventing health risks associated with the consumption of these products.

Despite the direct link between food products and obesity and NCDs, these excess nutritional components are not necessarily recognized by the different social sectors as harmful to health and are therefore no longer treated as such. However, public health institutions do recognize them and have been working to establish bilateral commitments with the food industry to reduce nutrients such as saturated fats, sugars and salt. However, effective regulation has not materialized, not least because of the Brazilian government's own difficulties in directly confronting market interests. The government then decided to adopt the strategy of formulating Cooperation Agreements between the parties, i.e. the Ministry of Health and a group of industry organizations. In the public institutions, the governance set up seemed to be an advance in democratic practice (public consultation, public hearing, regulatory agenda, etc.), but soon fell back with the advent of the Agreements. In this negotiation process, civil society - precisely the social segment most affected - was not involved, thus shaking the foundations of good governance.

The essence of this thesis focused on the discourses formulated by three groups of subjects investigated and linked to three different fields of activity: the market, public authorities and civil society. Based on their divergent positions on the health risks related to these products, they outlined different ways of regulating food risks. Those linked to the market defend the Agreement as a fair and correct alternative; those linked to public authorities are divided between defending the agreements and the need for compulsory rules and, finally, the representatives of civil society are unanimous in their defense of the regulatory measure (compulsory rules). As a result, the hypothesis formulated earlier[37] , has been confirmed in its initial part. There are not enough political forces to impose compulsory rules on industries to reduce nutrient levels within short timeframes and apply penalties in the event of non-compliance, with the aim of reformulating the nutritional composition of these products.

With regard to the complementary part of the hypothesis, the industry's approach to the problem of the relationship between food and NCDs was also confirmed. For the industry, the individual is responsible for risky behavior because they don't know how to choose food correctly and consume too much of it.

The recognition of the individual as a victim, due to the pressures of the fast pace of everyday life, the systematic inducements imposed by the food market through different mechanisms, and the omission of public control institutes, was practically obscured. Only the discourse of the market subject hinted at behavior that deviated from the market. This was the opposite of what happened with the civil society subjects, who emphasized the industry's share of responsibility.

At the same time as market players deny the fragility of the consumer in the face of the power of the market, they praise the food product as a source of life, health and longevity. For them, the possible risks that the products may carry are rare situations, given the set of control measures implemented by the industries themselves.

Based on the results of this thesis, it is possible to say that regulating food risks is a political arena where public demands are made in the midst of major disputes over

37 Hypothesis guiding the thesis: despite recognizing that public regulation of food is one of the necessary political-operational strategies to intervene in the emerging risks of food, the political forces in the current state are insufficient to implement it effectively, due to the power of the industries - which react by attributing responsibility for nutritional disorders to consumers and minimizing the demands of civil society.

interests. As neoliberal thinking grows stronger in the institutes of public power, and the market is placed on a level of superiority, the active participation of organized civil society becomes strategic for the effective defense of health interests. This participation by society, when legitimized, makes the link with the government so that it can fulfill its mission in defending public health issues.

By choosing to regulate the food market with the sole participation of this segment, the government has reduced its bargaining power and made itself more vulnerable to market demands. Organized civil society, if involved in this process of negotiation and agreement, would act as a counterpoint, since it is undoubtedly the representative that, in general, identifies and allies itself with the interests and needs of the people.

Guaranteeing healthy food is a citizen's right, a duty of the market and an object of control by the state. However, turning people into healthy citizens implies recognizing access to adequate food, health and nutrition as a fundamental right of every person. This requires respect for eating habits and practices and valuing people's health, among other aspects, so that everyone can fully exercise their citizenship.

In view of the above, it should be pointed out that in studies of this nature, involving a complex and multidimensional object of investigation, situated on the border of intersection between the socio-historical/current social, the national/international, the institutional/private, the political/technical and the physiological/symbolic, permeated by a thematic and value constellation, there are always limitations. Furthermore, such studies always involve a small number of subjects and target institutions, which means that the results represent only one version of the reality investigated. Recognizing the impact of all these interactions, in this study we have chosen to focus on the interactions (agreements and disagreements, demands and consents) of the institutional channels and private interests involved in regulating the food market to conform to a nutritious and healthier standard for all.

Finally, given the results of this thesis, the conceptual and strategic perspectives for the future could be as follows:

- Develop studies to assess the impact of the agreements formalized between this group of industry entities and the Ministry of Health, aimed at reducing nutrient levels, in this case sodium, on food products manufactured by companies that did not take part in the agreement. The alternative to "guaranteeing" that the many small and medium-sized food companies that did not take part in the negotiations would adhere to the proposal to adjust the nutritional profile of food would be to establish partnership or regulatory agreements. However, as the expectation of the Ministry of Health is that there will be a "cascade" effect after the agreement, which will trigger voluntary initiatives to reduce the sodium content of foods, it would be appropriate to prove this effect in specific studies;

- To explore the conceptual and practical bases of the Public-Private Partnership initiatives developed in the country in the field of nutrition, considering the conflicts of interest, the possibility of co-optation and intimidation of members of the government, demobilization to make compulsory rules viable, among other aspects that can arise from these partnerships. It will also investigate, from the point of view of public agents in the field of regulation, the impact of the initiative to formulate Agreements on current regulatory proposals;

- To evaluate the nutritional information initiatives and strategies, particularly those applied to food labels, being implemented in different countries. Then choose, in the light of the national socio-economic and cultural reality, those initiatives that present the most appropriate application to the Brazilian context, and;

- Broadening the dissemination of the risks of food and the diseases related to them, in spaces such as universities, schools, associations, class entities, trade unions and others, as a way of disseminating information, democratizing the debate and forming a social support base capable of opposing the rules imposed by the market with regard to the nutritional quality of food and food products placed on the market.

Finally, the Brazilian population cannot continue to be penalized in terms of their health and nutrition as a result of limited commitments signed between public institutions and the market. In the shadow of this penalization, there is a regulatory mechanism that remains open in the field of food risks. This is the main result expected from this study: to show that regulating does not only mean regulating the risks or nutritional components of food products. It involves the conflicts of interest linked to the production and marketing of these products; the subjective incorporation of the rules; and the management of resistance to the powers that impose them.

Regulation is never finished, but always ongoing, in the dynamic context of food risks. Similarly, there is no regulation without law, nor law without regulation, in the field of food control. Law and regulation are therefore an indispensable duo. However, regulation does not reside in the law, but precedes a need and mutual support in a regulatory process. It is the product of a collective invention, which updates rules and behaviors to give a new rationality to the practice of food control. In Brazilian institutions, the regulatory process has been established in a cooperative and democratic manner, except when there are no internal violations that deviate from these precepts.

In this sense, the aim of exploring the political, economic and subjective intricacies of regulating emerging food risks is to promote fair regulation. In other words, one that simultaneously and permanently creates the conditions for cooperative work, which implies the presence of the three key partners identified (the market, public authorities and civil society), particularly in such a culturally and symbolically sensitive sphere as this one. A conception of regulation that discards any instrumentalization of the process, with strict benefits for the interests of the market to legitimize it, but which is directed towards fair conduct at the service of society as a whole. Consent to such rules of fair conduct signals collaborative effectiveness and delimits the rights and duties of the three partners in the field in question.

BIBLIOGRAPHICAL REFERENCES

ALMEIDA, S.S.; NASCIMENTO, P.C.B.D.; QUAIOTI, T.C.B. Quantity and quality of food products advertised on Brazilian television. **Revista de Saùde Pùblica,** v.36, n.3, p.3535. 2002.

AMIGO, Hugo. Obesity in children in Latin America: situation, diagnostic criteria and challenges. **Cadernos de Saùblica**, v.19, sup.1, p.S163-S170, 2003.

ALTEKRUSE, S.F.; SWERDLOW, D.L. The changing epidemiology of foodborne diseases.

American Journal of the Medical Sciences. v.311, n.1, p.23-29, jan. 1996.

ANDRIEU, E.; DARMON, N.; DREWNOWSKI, A. Low-cost diets: more energy, fewer nutrients.

European Journal of Clinical Nutrition, v.60, p.434-436. 2006.

ARMSTRONG, G.L.; HOLLINGSWORTH, J.; GLENN MORRIS, J. Emerging Foodborne Pathogens: Escherichia coli O157:H7 as a Model of Entry of a New Pathogen into the Food Supply of the Developed World. **Epidemiologic Reviews,** v. 8, n.1, p.29-51, 1996.

BAKSHI, Anita. Potential adverse health effects of genetically modified crops. **Journal of Toxicology and Environmental Health**, Part B, v.6, p.211-225, 2003.

BARBOSA, A.O.; COSTA, E.A. The meanings of health security in the discourse of the National Health Surveillance Agency. **Ciência & Saùde Coletiva**, v. 15, n. Supl. 3, p.3361-3370. 2010.

BARDAL, P.A.P. et al. Current issues in the health surveillance of fluoride concentrations in food. **Cadernos de Saùde Pùblica**, Rio de Janeiro, v.28, n.3, p.573-582, mar. 2012.

BARROS, Diana Luz Pessoa de. **Teoria Semiótica do Texto**. 4. ed. 6. imp. Printed in the workshops of Editora Parma Ltda., 2005 Available at:

<http://copyfight.me/Acervo/livros/BARROS,%20Diana%20Luz%20Pessoa%20de%20- %20Teoria%20Semiotica%20do%20Texto.pdf >. Accessed on: June 15, 2014.

BARROS, M.B.A. et al. Trends in social and demographic inequalities in the prevalence of chronic diseases in Brazil, PNAD: 2003-2008. **Ciência & Saùde Coletiva**, v.16, n.9, p.3755-3768, 2011.

BATISTA FILHO, M.; RISSIN, A. The nutritional transition in Brazil: regional and temporal trends. **Cadernos de Saùde Pùblica**, Rio de Janeiro, v.19, sup. 1, p.S181-S191, 2003.

BAUMAN, Zygmunt. **Globalization: the human consequences.** Rio de Janeiro: Jorge Zahar Editor, 1999. 145p.

. **Life for consumption: the transformation of people into merchandise**. Rio de Janeiro: Jorge Zahar ed., 2008. 199p.

BEATON G.H.; MCHENRY, E.W. (eds), **Volume 3: Nutrition: a comprehensive treatise.** New York: Academic Press Inc, 1966.

BECK, Ulrich. **La sociedad del riesgo: hacia uma nueva modernidad.** Spain: PAIDÓS, 2002.

. **What is globalization? Equivocos do globalismo, resposta à globalizaçâ**. Sâo Paulo: Paz e Terra, 1999. 282p.

BEGHIN, J.C.; JENSEN, H.H. Farm policies and added sugar in Us diets. **Food Policy,** v.33, p.480-488, 2008.

BERGER , P. L.; LUCKMANN, T. **The social construction of reality.** 31. ed. Petrópolis, RJ: Vozes Ltda., 2009.

BERMUDEZ, O. I.; TUCKER, K. L. Trends in dietary patterns of Latin American populations. **Cadernos de Saùde Pùblica**, Rio de Janeiro, v.19, sup. 1, p.S87-S99, 2003.

BEZERRA, I. N.; et al. Out-of-home food consumption in Brazil. **Revista de Saùde Pùblica**, Sâo Paulo, v. 47, Supl. 1, p.200S-11S, 2013. Available at:

<ww.scielo.br/pdf/rsp/v47s1/06.pdf>. Accessed on: 26 Nov. 2014.

BLEIL, Suzana Inez. The Western Food Pattern: considerations on changing habits in Brazil. UNICAMP **Revista Cadernos de Debate**. v. 6, p.1-25, 1998.

BOBBIO, Norberto. **State, government and society: towards a general theory of politics**. 12. ed. Rio de Janeiro: Paz e Terra, 2005.

BODSTEIN, Regina Cele de Andrade. he complexity of the contemporary social order and the redefinition of public responsibility. In: Rozenfeld, S. (org). **Fundamentals of Health Surveillance**. Rio de Janeiro: Ed. Fiocruz, p.63-97, 2000.

BORCH, A; ROOS, G. Public Private Partnerships fighting obesity in Europe ", **Anthropology of food** [Online], S7 | 2012. Available at: <URL: <http://aof.revues.org/7286>. Accessed on: June 26, 2014.

BOUCHRIF, B. et al. Prevalence and antibiotic-resistance of Salmonella isolated from food in Morocco. **The Journal of Infection in Developing Countries**, v.3, n.1, p.35-40, 2009.

BOURDIEU, Pierre. **Symbolic power.** Rio de Janeiro: Bertrand Brasil, 2009.

. **Counterfires: for a European social movement**. Rio de Janeiro: Jorge Zahar ed., 2001. 115p.

BRANCA, F; NIKOGOSIAN, H; LOBSTEIN ,T (ed). **The challenge of obesity in the WHO European Region and the strategies for response: summary.** Copenhagen, Denmark: WHO Library Cataloguing in Publication Data, 2007.

BRAZIL. **Decree-Law No. 986 of October 21, 1969.** Available at:

<http://portal.anvisa.gov.br/wps/wcm/connect/836d7c804745761d8415d43fbc4c6735/ dec_lei_986.pdf?MOD=AJPERES.>. Accessed on: April 15, 2014.

. **Law n. 9.782, of January 26, 1999**. Defines the National Health Surveillance System, creates the National Health Surveillance Agency, and makes other provisions.

Available at: <http://www.planalto.gov.br/ccivil_03/leis/l9782.htm>. Accessed on: 23 Feb. 2014.

National Health Surveillance Agency. **Resolution - RDC No. 28, of March 28, 2000.** Provides for the basic procedures for Good Manufacturing Practices in establishments that process salt for human consumption and the roadmap for sanitary inspections in salt-processing factories. Available at: <http://189.28.128.100/nutricao/docs/legislacao/resolucaordc_28.pdf>. Accessed on: April 25, 2014.

. **Resolution - RDC No. 40, of March 21, 2001**. To approve the Technical Regulation for Compulsory Nutritional Labeling of Packaged Foods and Beverages, set out in the Annex to this Resolution.

. **Resolution - RDC No. 344, of December 13, 2002.** To approve the Technical Regulation for the Fortification of Wheat Flour and Corn Flour with Iron and Folic Acid, set out in the Annex to this Resolution. Official Journal of the Union; Executive Branch, December 18, 2002. Available at: <http://portal.anvisa.gov.br/wps/wcm/connect/f851a500474580668c83dc3fbc4c6735/R DC_344_2002.pdf?MOD=AJPERES.>. Accessed on: April 25, 2014.

. Controlling the addition of iodine to salt reduces cases of goiter. **Boletim Informativo,** n.41, p. 4-5, Mar. 2004. Available at:

<http://www.anvisa.gov.br/divulga/public/boletim/41_04.pdf.>. Accessed on: April 20, 2014.

. **Advisory Board.** 2005 (?). Agency/Publication Agency. Anvisa Portal. Available at:< http://s.anvisa.gov.br/wps/s/r/9xd.>. Accessed on: 28 Apr. 2014.

. **Ordinance No. 354, of August 11, 2006a.** (Republished in the DOU of 21.08.06 and rectified in the DOU of 29.08.06). Approves and promulgates the Internal Regulations of the National Health Surveillance Agency - ANVISA and makes other provisions.

. **Public Consultation No. 71, of November 10, 2006b**. Official Gazette of November 13, 2006. Approve the regulation on the offer, advertising, publicity, information and other related practices aimed at publicizing and promoting foods considered to have high amounts of sugar, saturated fat, *trans* fat, sodium, and drinks with low nutritional content. Available at:

<http://www.anvisa.gov.br/propaganda/minuta_consulta71_2006.pdf>. Accessed on: 28 Apr. 2014.

. **Management 2005-2010: main achievements**. National Health Surveillance Agency. Brasilia: Anvisa, 2010a.

. **Resolution-RDC No. 24, of June 15, 2010b**. Provides for the offer, advertising, publicity, information and other related practices whose purpose is the dissemination and commercial promotion of foods considered to have high amounts of sugar, saturated fat, *trans* fat, sodium, and beverages with low nutritional content, under the terms of this Resolution, and makes other provisions. Available at: < http://portal.anvisa.gov.br/wps/wcm/connect/345653804745975 49fd4df3fbc4c6735 /RD C24 10 Publicidade+de+alimentos.pdf?MOD=AJPERES>. Accessed on April 28, 2014.

. **Nutritional profile of processed foods**. Technical Report No. 42/2010c. Available at: <www.anvisa.gov.br/wpm/connect/1011330044bbafc3b1f6b10377ff0da5/Perfil+Nutr icio nal.pdf?MOD=AJPERES>. Accessed on: 22 Nov. 2010.

. **Program for the Analysis of Pesticide Residues in Food (PARA).** 2010 Activity Report General Toxicology Management. Brasilia, December 5, 2011. Available at: <http://portal.anvisa.gov.br/wps/wcm/connect/b380fe004965d38ab6abf74ed75891a e/R elat%C3%B3rio+PARA+2010+-+Vers%C3%A3o+Final.pdf?MOD=AJPERES>. Accessed on:04 nov. 2013.

. Guidance document. **Regulatory agenda. Four-year cycle 2013-2016.** Anvisa's

Good Regulatory Practices Program. Brasilia:Anvisa, 2012 Available at: <file:///Users/anavirginiafigueiredo/Documents/ATESE/CAPITULOS%20DA%20TESE /RE GULACAO/Agenda_Regulatoria_Quadrienal_final_baixa.pdf>. Accessed on: 27 Apr. 2014.

. **Topics on the regulatory agenda. 2013-2014 BIENNIUM**. Complete list and progress of topics, March 2014. Regulatory Agenda Quadrennial Cycle 2013-2016. Available at:

<http://portal.anvisa.gov.br/wps/wcm/connect/c4a4840043684e988946ed74bfb0241 1/ Proposta_Completa_Temas_30_setembro.pdf?MOD=AJPERES>. Accessed on: 27 Apr. 2014.

. Civil House. Infrastructure Chamber - Economic Policy Chamber. **Report of the Interministerial Working Group Analysis and Evaluation of the Role of Regulatory Agencies in the Current Brazilian Institutional Arrangement**. Report of the Interministerial Working Group. Brasilia, September 2003. Available at:

<http://www.bresserpereira.org.br/Documents/MARE/Agencias/avaliacao_das_agenci as_r eguladoras_-_casa_civil.pdf.>. Accessed on: February 20, 2014.

Chamber of Deputies. Internal Rules of the Chamber of Deputies. 11. ed. Brasilia, 2013. Available at:

<file:///Users/anavirginiafigueiredo/Downloads/regimento interno 11ed.pdf.>. Accessed on: May 15, 2014.

. National Council of Health Secretaries. Law No. 8080, of September 19, 1990. In:. **Legislaçâo do SUS**. Brasilia:CONASS, p.22-37. 2003a.

.. Federal Constitution 1988, Title VIII, Social Order, Section II Health.

In:. **Legislaçâo do SUS**. Brasilia:CONASS, p.20-21. 2003b.

. Law 9782, of January 26, 1999. Defines the National Health Surveillance System, creates the National Health Surveillance Agency and makes other provisions. In:. **Legislaçâo do SUS.** Brasilia:CONASS, p.169-181. 2003c.

. National Council for Food and Nutrition Security. WG - Adequate and Healthy Food. **Final Report.** March 2007. Available at:

<http://www4.planalto.gov.br/consea/documentos/alimenatacao-adequada-e-saudavel/documento-final-alimentacao-adequada-e-saudavel>. Accessed on: March 15,

2012.

. Brazilian Institute of Geography and Statistics. **Family Budget Survey, 2008-2009. Anthropometry and Nutritional Status of Children, Adolescents and Adults in Brazil.** Rio de Janeiro, 2010. Available at: http://portal.saude.gov.br/portal/arquivos/pdf/pof_2008_2009_encaa.pdf. Accessed on: March 11, 2012.

. Family Budget Survey, 2008-2009. **Analysis of Food Consumption in Brazil**. Rio de Janeiro: IBGE, 2011.

. National Institute of Metrology, Quality and Technology. *Codex Alimentarius* Committee of Brazil - CCAB. **History of the *Codex Alimentarius* Committee of Brazil - CCAB**. Website http://www.inmetro.gov.br/index.asp. Available at:

<http://www.inmetro.gov.br/qualidade/comites/codex_ccab.asp>. Accessed on: April 16, 2014.

. Ministry of Social Development and Fight against Hunger. Executive Secretariat of the Interministerial Chamber for Food and Nutritional Security - CAISAN. **Intersectoral Plan for the Prevention and Control of Obesity**. Press release. Estimated year 2012a. Available at:

<http://www4.planalto.gov.br/consea/noticias/documentos/planalto-intersetorial-de-prevention-and-control-of-obesity>. Accessed on: April 28, 2014.

. Food and Nutrition Education Reference Framework for Public Policies. Brasilia, DF:MDS; National Secretariat for Food and Nutrition Security, 2012b.

;;Ministry of Health. **Evaluation of the temporal evolution of the nutritional status of children between 0 and 5 years of age who are beneficiaries of the Bolsa Familia Program (PBF), accompanied by health conditionalities. Executive Summary**. Brasilia, April 2014. Available at:

<http://aplicacoes.mds.gov.br/sagirmps/simulacao/sum executivo/pdf/sumario 138.pdf> . Accessed on: June 18, 2014.

. Ministry of Health. **8ª National Health Conference**. Brasilia-DF, March 17-21, 1986. Available at:

<http://bvsms.saude.gov.br/bvs/publicacoes/8_conferencia_nacional_saude_relatorio_f inal .pdf.> Accessed on:17 Mar. 2014.

. **Ordinance No. 710, of June 10, 1999**. Approves the National Food and Nutrition Policy, the full text of which is set out in the annex to this ordinance. Diàrio Oficial da Uniâo; Poder Executivo, June 15, 1999.

. **Health in Mercosur**. - 2. ed. rev. and ampl., 1.≡ reprint. - Brasilia: Ministério da Saùde, 2003 24 p.: il. - (Series B. Textos Bàsicos de Saùde). Available at: <http://dtr2001.saude.gov.br/editora/produtos/livros/pdf/03_0401_M.pdf.>. Accessed on: December 10, 2013.

. Secretariat for Labor Management and Health Education. Department of Health Work Management and Regulation. **Mercosur permanent forum for health work**. Brasilia: Ministry of Health, 2007a. (Series D. Meetings and Conferences) Available at: <http://bvsms.saude.gov.br/bvs/publicacoes/forum_permanente_mercosul_trabalho_sa ud e.pdf>. Accessed on: Dec. 10, 2013.

. **Ordinance No. 3.092, of December 4, 2007b**. Establishes a Technical Group with the aim of discussing and proposing joint actions to be implemented to improve the supply of food products and promote healthy eating. Available at: <http://dtr2001.saude.gov.br/sas/PORTARIAS/Port2007/GM/GM-3092.htm>. Accessed on: April 28, 2014.

. **It deals with the Ministry of Health's agreement with the Brazilian Association of Food Industries to reduce the sodium, fat and sugar content of foods.** Estimated year 2007c. Available at: http://189.28.128.100/nutricao/docs/geral/acordo_social_reducao_teores_sodio_acuca r_g orduras.pdf. Accessed on: March 15, 2012.

. **Strategic Action Plan to Combat Chronic Non-Communicable Diseases (NCDs) in Brazil - 2011-2022**. Ministry of Health. Health Surveillance Secretariat. Department of Health Situation Analysis. Brasilia: Ministry of Health, 2011. 148p. (Series B. Textos Bàsicos de Saùde).

. **National food and nutrition policy.** Preliminary version. 2012a. Available at: http://189.28.128.100/nutricao/docs/geral/pnan2011.pdf. Accessed on: March 25, 2012.

. **Vigitel Brazil 2011: Estimates of the frequency and sociodemographic distribution of risk and protective factors for chronic diseases in the capitals of the 26 Brazilian states and the Federal District in 2011**. Ministério da Saùde, Secretaria de Vigilância em Saùde - Brasilia: Ministério da Saùde, 2012b. (Series G. Statistics and Health Information).

Building the reformulation agenda for processed foods with the food industries. 30 Apr. 2012c. Available:

http://nutricao.saude.gov.br/sodio_reformulacao.php>. Accessed on: June 24, 2014.

. **Vigitel Brazil 2012.Surveillance of risk and protective factors for chronic diseases by telephone survey. Estimates of the frequency and sociodemographic distribution of risk and protective factors for chronic diseases in the capitals of the 26 Brazilian states and the Federal District in 2012**. Brasilia: Ministry of Health. 2013.

Available at: <http://www.sbpt.org.br/downloads/arquivos/vigitel_2012.pdf>. Accessed on: 01 Mar.2014.

. **Vigitel Brazil 2013. Surveillance of risk and protective factors for chronic diseases by telephone survey. Estimates of the frequency and sociodemographic distribution of risk and protective factors for chronic diseases in the capitals of the 26 Brazilian states and the Federal District in 2013.** Brasilia-DF/Ministry of Health. 2014a.

Available at:< http://biavati.files.wordpress.com/2014/05/vigitel-2013.pdf>. Accessed on: June 15, 2014.

. **Reduction of Sodium, Sugar and *Trans* Fat Promotion of Health and Adequate and Healthy Nutrition.** 2014b. Available at:

<http://dab.saude.gov.br/portaldab/ape_promocao_da_saude.php?conteudo=reducao.> Accessed on: June 23, 2014.

Presidency of the Republic**. Constitutional Amendment No. 64, of February 4, 2010**. Available at:

<http://www.planalto.gov.br/ccivil 03/constituicao/Emendas/Emc/emc64.htm>. Accessed on Aug. 10, 2014.

BAUM, Fran. Health, equity, justice and globalization: some lessons from the People's Health Assembly. **Journal of Epidemiology & Community Health**, v.55, p.613-616. 2001.

BRESSER PEREIRA, Luis Carlos G. Reflexoes sobre a reforma gerencial brasileira de 1995. **Revista do Serviço Pùblico.** ano 50 n.4, Oct-Dec. p.5-29, 1999.

. The structural model of public management. **Revista de Administraçâo Pùblica** . Rio de Janeiro, v.42, n.2, p.391-410, mar./abr. 2008.

BUCHLER, S.; SMITH, K.; LAWRENCE, G. Food risks, old and new: demographic characteristics and perceptions of food additives, regulation and contamination in AustraliaJournal of Sociology. **The Australian Sociological Association**, v.46, n.4 p.353374, 2010.

BURBANO, J. C.; FORNASINI, M.; ACOSTA, M. Prevalence and factors of overweight in schoolgirls aged 12 to 19 in a semi-urban region of Ecuador. **Revista Panamericana de Salud Publica**, v.13, n.5, p.227-284, 2003.

CABALLERO, Benjamin. The global epidemic of obesity: an overview. **Epidemiologic Reviews,** v.29, n.1, p.1-5, 2007.

CANESQUI, A.M.; GARCIA, R.M.D. An introduction to reflection on the sociocultural approach to food. In: (eds). **Anthropology and nutrition: a possible dialog.** Rio de Janeiro: Editora FIOCRUZ, p.9-19. 2005.

CARAPINHEIRO, Graça. The globalization of social risk. In: SANTOS, B DE S (org). **A** globalizaçâo **e as ciências sociais**. 2≡ Ed. Sâo Paulo: Cortez, ch. 5, p.197-228, 2002.

CARVALHEIRO, José da Rocha. Challenges of Health Surveillance and the Regulatory Function. In: BRAZIL. Ministry of Health. **1st National Health Surveillance Conference: Textbooks**. Brasilia: National Health Surveillance Agency, p.25-36. 2001.

CASTEL, Robert. From dangerousness to risk. In: BURCHELL, G.; GRAHAM, C.; MILLER, P. (eds.). **The Foucault effect: studies in governmentality**. Chicago: The University of Chicago Press. p.281-299, 1991.

CHANDON, P.; WANSINK , B. Does food marketing need to make us fat? A review and solutions. **Nutrition** Reviews, v.70, n.10, p.571-593. 2012. Available at:

<file:///Users/anavirginiafigueiredo/Documents/ATESE/CAPITULOS%20DA%20TESE /DI ETA_CONSUMO/national_capacity_prevention_ncds.pdf>. Accessed on: 06 Mar.2014.

CHAVES, Nelson. **Nutrition: basic and applied.** Rio de Janeiro: Editora Guanabara Koogan SA, 1978. 344p.

CHOPRA, Mickey. Globalization and food: implications for the promotion of "healthy" diets. In: WORLD HEALTH ORGANIZATION. **Globalization diets and noncommunicable diseases.** Switzerland: WHO Library, p.1-16. 2002.

CHOPRA, M; GALBRAITH, S & DARNTON-HILL, I. A global response to a global problem: the epidemic of overnutrition. **Bulletin of the World Health Organization**, v.80, p.12, p.952958, 2002.

CONTRERAS, Jesús Hernàndez. Food modernity between overabundance and insecurity. **International Journal of Sociology**. Tercera Epoca, n.40. p. 109-132, ene./abr. 2005.

.; GRACIA, M. **Alimentaçâo, sociedade e cultura**. Rio de Janeiro: Editora Fiocruz, 2011.

COSTA, Edinà Alves. **Health surveillance: protecting and defending health.** Sao Paulo: Hucitec, 1999. 460p.

. Regulation and health surveillance for health protection. In: Vieira, F. P.;

REDIGUIERI, C. F.; REDIGUIERI, C.F. (eds). **A Regulaçâo de Medicamentos no Brasil, Porto Alegre:** Editora: ARTMED; p.21-37. 2013.

COSTA, N.R et al. O desenho institucional da reforma regulatória e as falhas de mercado no setor saùde. **Revista da Administraçâo Pùblica**, Rio de Janeiro, v. 35, n.2, p.193:228, mar./abr. 2001.

COSTA, R.F.; CINTRA, I.P.; FISBERG, M. Prevalence of overweight and obesity in schoolchildren in the city of Santos, SP. **Arquivos Brasileiros de Endocrinologia e Metabologia**, v.50, n.1, p.60-67, feb. 2006.

COUTINHO, J.G.; GENTIL, P.C.; TORAL, N.A. malnutrition and obesity in Brazil: tackling them based on the single nutrition agenda. **Cadernos de Saùblica**, v.24, sup. 2, p.S332-S340, 2008.

CRESWELL, John W. **Research design: qualitative, quantitative and mixed methods.** 3. ed. Porto Alegre: Artmed, 2010.

CRUZ, Verônica. State and regulation: theoretical foundations. In: RAMALHO, P.I.S. (org).

Regulation and regulatory agencies: governance and regulatory impact analysis. la ed. Brasila: Anvisa, , p. 53-86, 2009.

DEL GROSSI, M.D. Poverty reduction: From 44 million to 29.6 million People. In: GRAZIANO DA SILVA, J; DEL GROSSI, M. E.; FRANÇA, C. G. (orgs.) **The Fome Zero (Zero Hunger) Program: The Brazilian experience.** Brasilia: MDA, 2010. Available at: <http://www.fao.org/docrep/016/i3023e/i3023e.pdf.>. Accessed on: October 18, 2013.

DIETZ, William H. Critical periods in childhood for the development of obesity. **American Journal Clinical Nutrition**, v.59, n.5, p.955-59, may, 1994.

DAHLET, Patrick. Written production, cognitive and textual approaches. Applied linguistic work. IEL Unicamp:Campinas, v. 23, p.79-95, jan./jul. 1994.

. Erasing divisions, celebrating consensus: discursive governance in the neoliberal era. Todas as letras w, Sâo Paulo, v.16, n.1, p.125-138, mai. 2014. Disponivel em: <http:dx.doi.org/10.15529/1980.6914/letras.v16n1p125-138.>. Accessed on: July 22, 2014.

DELORMIER, T.; FROHLICH, K. L.; POTVIN, L. Food and eating as social practice - understanding eating patterns as social phenomena and implications for public health.

Sociology of Health & Illness, v. 31, n. 2, p. 215-228, 2009.

DOAK, C.M. et al. Overweight and underweight coexist within households in Brazil, China and Russia. **Journal of Nutrition**, v.130, n.12, p.2965-2971, dec., 2000.

DREWNOWSKI, Adam. Fat and sugar: an economic analysis **Journal of Nutrition**, v.133, n.3, p.838S-840S, mar. 1. 2003.

Intense sweeteners and energy density of foods: implications for weight control. **European Journal of Clinical Nutrition**, v.53, p.757-763. 1999.

. Obesity, diets, and social inequalities. **Nutrition Reviews.** v. 67, sup. 1, p.S36-S39. 2009.

. The cost of US foods as related to their nutritive value. **American Journal of Clinical Nutrition,** v.92, p.1181-8. 2010.

et al. Dietary Energy Density and Body Weight: Is There a Relationship? **Nutrition Reviews**, v. 62, n. 11, p. 403-413, nov. 2004.

POPKIN, B.M. The Nutrition Transition: New Trends in the Global Diet. **Nutrition Reviews**, v. 55, n. 2, p.31-43, feb. 1997.

.; SPECTER, S.E. Poverty and obesity: the role of energy density and energy costs.

American Journal of Clinical Nutrition, v.79, n.1, p.6-16, jan. 2004.

EVANS, M. et al Globalization, diet, and health: an example from Tonga. **Bulletin of the World Health Organization**, v.79, n.9, p. 856-862, 2001.

EWALD, François. Insurance and risk. In: BURCHELL, G.; GRAHAM, C.; MILLER, P. (eds.). **The Foucault effect: studies in governmentality**. Chicago: The University of Chicago Press. p.197-210, 1991.

EGGER, G.; SWINBURN, B. An "ecological" approach to the obesity pandemic. **British Medical Journal**. v.315, n. 23, aug. 1997. Available at:

<http://www.ncbi.nlm.nih.gov/pmc/articles/PMC2127317/pdf/9284671.pdf>. Accessed on: 26 Nov. 2014.

FOOD AND AGRICULTURE ORGANIZATION OF UNITED NATIONS. Report of The eighteenth session of The Committee on agriculture. Rome 9-10 february 2004. **FAO's Proposed Follow-up to the Report of Joint WHO/FAO Expert Consultation on Diet, Nutrition and the Prevention of Chronic Diseases .** 2004.

. **Application of risk analysis to food standards issues: report of the FAO/WHO mixed expert consultation**. Geneva, Switzerland, March 13-17, 1995. WHO/FNU/FOS/95.3. Available at: <http://www.fao.org/3/a-x1271s.pdf.> Accessed on: 07 Mar. 2013.

. Globalization of food systems in developing countries: impact on food security and nutrition. **FAO Food Nutrition Paper 83.** 2004, Reprinted 2006.

. **Responding to the food crisis: synthesis of medium-term measures proposed in inter-agency assessments.** ROME, 2009. Available at:

<http://www.fao.org/fileadmin/user_upload/ISFP/SR_Web.pdf>. Accessed on: March 21, 2012.

. **World hunger is decreasing, but remains unacceptably high: The objectives of the international community in reducing hunger are difficult to achieve**. Economic and Social Department September 2010.

. **FAO in the 21st century; ensuring food security in a changing world**.

FAO:Rome, 2011a.

. **The state of food insecurity in the world: How does international price volatility affect domestic economies and food security?** FAO:Rome, 2011b.

. **Sustainable nutrition security: Restoring the bridge between agriculture and health**. Rome: FAO, Sept. 2012.

. **Fao statistical yearbook 2013**. World Food and Agriculture, Rome:FAO, 2013a. Available at: http://www.fao.org/docrep/018/i3107e/i3107e.PDF>. Accessed on: 17 Nov. 2014.

. **The state of food and agriculture: food systems for better nutrition**, Rome, 2013b.

;_WORLD HEALTH ORGANIZATION. *Codex Alimentarius Commission.* **Manual of Procedures.** Joint FAO/WHO Program on Food Standards. *14-* ed. Rome. 2005.

FAO; WHO. **Request for comments on draft action plan for implementation of the global strategy on diet, physical activity and health**. CL 2006/44-CACSeptember 2006a. Available at: <ftp://ftp.fao.org/codex/Circular_Letters/CxCL2006/cl06_44e.pdf>. Accessed on: June 3, 2014.

. **Undestanding Codex Alimentarius.** Third edition. Issued by the Secretariat of the Joint FAO/WHO Food Standards Programme, FAO, Rome. 2006b. Available at: <ftp://ftp.fao.org/codex/Publications/understanding/Understanding_EN.pdf>. Accessed on: 13 Nov. 2013.

. Joint Fao/Who Food Standards Program .Codex Alimentarius Commission. Thirty Fifth Session Rome, Italy, July 2-7, 2012. **Report of the fortieth session of the Codex Committee on food labeling.** Ottawa, Canada 15 - 18 May 2012. Available at: <ftp://ftp.fao.org/codex/Reports/Reports_2012/REP12_FLe.pdf>. Accessed on: July 3, 2014.

. Agenda Item 2(A) Cx/Nfsdu 13/35/2 Joint Fao/Who Food Standards Programme Codex Committee on Nutrition and Foods for Special Dietary Uses .Thirty-fifth Session Bad Soden am Taunus, Germany 4 - 8 November 2013. **Matters Referred to the Committee by the Codex Alimentarius Commission and/or Other Codex Committees.** Available at: <ftp://ftp.fao.org/codex/Meetings/ccnfsdu/ccnfsdu35/nf35_02e.pdf>. Accessed on: July 3, 2014.

FERNANDEZ SAN JUAN, P.M. Dietary habits and nutritional status of school aged children in Spain. **Nutrición Hospitalaria**, v.21, n.3, p.374-378, 2006.

FERREIRA, V.A. et al. Inequality, poverty and obesity. **Ciência & Saùde Coletiva**, v.15, supl. 1, p.1423-1432, 2010.

FIGUEIREDO, A.V.A. ; MIRANDA, M.S. Risk analysis applied to food in Brazil: perspectives and challenges. **Ciência & Saùde Coletiva**, v.16, n.4, p.2251-2262, 2011.

FISCHLER, Claude. Food, Self and Identity. **Social Science Information,** v.27, p.275293,1988.

FLICK, Uwe. Introduction to qualitative research. 3 ed., Porto Alegre: Ed Artmed, 2009.

FOUCAULT, Michel. **Microphysics of power.** 3.ed., Rio de Janeiro: Ediçôes Graal Ltda, 1982. 295p.

. **The order of discourse.** 5.ed. Sâo Paulo: Ediçôes Loyola. 1999. 79p.

. **Archaeology of knowledge.** 7. ed. Rio de Janeiro: Forense University. 2008. 236p.

FREIRE, Paulo. Education as the practice of freedom. Rio de Janeiro: Paz e Terra, 2010.

GARCIA, Rosa Wanda Diez. Reflexes of globalization on food culture: considerations on changes in urban eating. **Revista de Nutriçâo**, Campinas, 16(4):483-492, Oct./Dec, 2003.

GRACIA, Maria Arnaiz. Towards a New Food Order? In: CANESQUI, A.M.;

GARCIA, R.W.D. (eds). **Anthropology and Nutrition: a possible dialog.** Rio de Janeiro: Editora Fiocruz, 2005, p.147-164.

. Eating well, eating badly: the medicalization of eating behavior. **Salud Pùblica,** México. n.49, v.3, p.236-242.,may/jun. 2007.

GIDDENS, Anthony. **The consequences of modernity.** Translated by Raul Fiker. Sâo Paulo: Ed. UNESP, 1991.

. **Sociology.** 6- ed. Lisbon: Calouste Gulbenkian Foundation; 2008.

. **The world in the age of globalization**. Lisbon: Editorial Presença, 7. ed. 2010.

GOMES, Eduardo Granha Magalhâes. Independent regulatory agencies and the TCU: conflict of jurisdictions? **Revista de Administraçâo Pùblica**, v.40, n.4, p.615-30, jul/ago. 2006.

GONÇALVES, Alcindo. The concept of governance. In : CONPEDI, VIV., 2005, Fortaleza. **National Meeting of the National Council for Research and Postgraduate Studies in Law.** - CONPEDI. Fortaleza: Boiteux Foundation, 2005. Available at:

<http://conpedi.org.br/manaus/arquivos/anais/XIVCongresso/078.pdf>. Accessed on: 27 Mar. 2014.

GREIMAS, Algirdas Julien. **Du Sens,** ed. Le Seuil, 1970.

GUTIÉRREZ-FISAC, J.L et al. The obesity epidemic and its related factors: the case of Spain. Cad. Saùde Pùblica, Rio de Janeiro, 19(Suppl. 1):S101-S110, 2003.

HALKIER, Bente Risk and food: environmental concerns and consumer practices.

International Journal of Food Science and Technology, v.36, p.801-812, 2001.

HALL, G.V.; D'SOUZA, R.M.; KIRK, M.D. Foodborne disease in the new millennium: out of the frying pan and into the fire? **Medical Journal of Australia**, v.177, n. 2/16, p.614-618, dec., 2002.

HARRIS, J.L et al. A crisis in the marketplace: How food marketing contributes to childhood obesity and what can be done. **Annual Review of Public Health**, v.30, p.211-25, 2009.

HASTINGS, G. et al. Review of research on the effects of food promotion to children. Final Report. 22nd September 2003. Executive Summary. The University of Strathclyde.

Available at: <http://www.food.gov.uk/multimedia/ pdfs/promofoodchildrenexec.pdf>. Accessed on: March 28, 2010.

. The extent, nature and effects of food promotion to children: A review of the evidence. In: Marketing of food and non-alcoholic beverages to children: report of a WHO forum and technical meeting. Oslo, Norway, May 2-5, 2006. Geneva, Switzerland. WHO Press.

HAWKES, Corinna. Marketing Activities of Global Soft Drink and Fast Food Companies in Emerging Markets: a Review. IN: WHO.**Globalization, Diets and Noncommunicable Diseases**. Geneva/Switzerland:WHO Library Cataloguing-in-Publication Data. 2002.

. **Food marketing to children: the global regulatory landscape.** Brasilia: Pan American Health Organization; National Health Surveillance Agency, 2006.

. Regulation food marketing to young people worldwide: trends and policy drives. **American Journal of Public Health,** v.97, n.11, p.1962-1973, 2007.

. Dietary Implications of Supermarket Development: A Global Perspective.

Development Policy Review, v.26, n.6, p.657-69. 2008a.

. High Level Group Working Paper on Public Private Partnerships for Health. 2008b. Available at:

<ec.europa.eu/health/ph_determinants/life_style/nutrition/documents/ev20081028_wp_e n.pdf>. Accessed on: July 23, 2014.

. Public health sector and food industry interaction: it's time to clarify the term 'patnership'and be honest about underlying interests. **European Journal of Public Health**, v.21, n4, 400-403. 2011. Available at: <http://eurpub.oxfordjournals.org>.

Accessed on: Nov. 11, 2013.

HENDERSON, J. et al. What are the important issues around food safety and nutrition? Findings from a media analysis and qualitative study of consumer trust. **Australasian Medical Journal,** v.1, n.2, 164-169, 2010.

HESPANHA, Pedro. Malaise and social risk in a globalized world: new problems and new challenges for social theory. In: SANTOS, B.S. (org). **A** globalizaçâo **e as ciências sociais.** 2≡ Ed. Sâo Paulo: Cortez, ch.4, p.161-196, 2002.

HUTIN, Y.J.F et al.. A Multistate, Foodborne outbreak of Hepatitis A. **The New England Journal of Medicine,** v.340, n. 8, p. 595-602, feb. 1999.

BRAZILIAN INSTITUTE OF SOCIAL AND ECONOMIC ANALYSIS. **Repercussoes do Programa Bolsa Familia na segurança alimentar e nutricional: relatório sintese.** Rio de Janeiro: iBAsE, 2008.

IANNI, Octavio. **The age of globalization.** 9≡ ed., Rio de Janeiro: Civilizaçâo Brasileira, 2007. 252p.

KAiN, J.; Vio, F.; ALBALA, c. obesity trends and determinant factors in Latin America. **Cadernos de Saùde Pùblica,** v.19, sup.1, p.S77-S86, 2003

KAFERSTEIN, EK; MOTARJEMI, Y & BETTCHER , DW. Foodborne Disease Control: A Transnational Challenge. **Emerging Infectious Diseases**, v. 3, n. 4, p.503-10, oct./dec. 1997.

KATZ, D. et al. Cyclosporiasis associated with imported raspberries Florida, 1996. **Public Health Reports**, v.114:427-38, sep./oct. 1999.

KENNEDY, G.; NANTEL, G.; SHETTY, P. Globalization of food systems in developing countries: a synthesis of country case studies 1 FAO Food and Nutrition paper n. 83. Rome:FAO, 2004. Available at: <http://www.fao.org/3/a-y5736e/>. Accessed on: May 15, 2014.

KING, L.A. et al. Community-wide outbreak of Escherichia coli 0157:H7 associated with consumption of frozen beef burgers. **Epidemiology and Infection,** p.889-896, 2009.

KIRK, M.D. et al. An outbreak due to peanuts in their shell caused by Salmonella enterica serotypes Stanley and Newport - sharing molecular information to solve international outbreaks. **Epidemiology & Infection,** v.132, p.571-577, 2004.

LABONTÉ, R; MOHINDRA, K & LECUCHA, R. Framing international trade and chronic disease. **Globalization and Health**, v.7, n.21, p.1-15, 2011.

LANG, Tim.The complexities of globalization: The UK as a case study of tensions within the food system and the challenge to food policy. **Agriculture and Human Values**, v.16, p.169185, 1999.

LUCCHESE, Geraldo A. Internationalization of health regulation. **Ciências e saùde coletiva,** v.8, n.2, p.537-555, 2003.

. **Globalization and health regulation: the direction of health surveillance in Brazil**. Brasilia: Anvisa, 2008.

LUHMANN, Niklas. **Risk: a sociological theory.** New York: Wlater de Gruyter Inc., 1993.

LUPTON, Deborah A. Lay discourses and beliefs related to food risks: an Australian perspective. **Sociology of Health & Illness**, v.27 No. 4, p. 448-467, 2005.

MACIEL, Maria E.unice. Cultural Identity and Food. In: CANESQUI, A.M.; GARCIA, R.W.D. (eds). **Anthropology and Nutrition: a possible dialog**. Rio de Janeiro: Editora Fiocruz, 2005. p.49-55.

MAJONE, Giandomenico. From the positive state to the regulatory state: causes and consequences of the change in the mode of governance. Economic Regulation and Democracy: The European Debate.

São Paulo: Editora Singular, 2006. Available at: <http://academico.direito-rio.fgv.br/ccmw/images/0/08/Majone.pdf>. Accessed on: March 10, 2014.

MALUF, Renato. **Food and Nutritional Security.** Petrópolis: Editora Vozes, 2007.

; MENEZES, F; VALENTE, F.L. Contribution to the theme of food security in Brazil. **Cadernos de Debate**, p.4:66-88, 1996.

MARINHO S. P. et al. Obesity in adults from impoverished segments. **Revista de Nutriçâo**, v.16, n.2, p.195-201, apr./jun., 2003.

MARTINS, I. S. et al. Poverty, malnutrition and obesity; interrelation of nutritional status of individuals from the same family. **Ciência e saùde coletiva**, v.12, n.6, p.1553-1565, nov./dez., 2007.

MAZZOCCHI, M; SHANKAR, B.; TRAILL, B. The development of global diets since icn 1992: influences of agri-food sector trends and policies. Food Commodity and Trade Policy Research Working Paper n. 34. Rome:FAO, october, 2012.

MCDERMOTT, L.; STEAD, M.; HASTINGS, G. A marketing strategy to review the effects of food promotion to children. Case Study 4. 30 mar. 2007. Available at: <http://www.stir.ac.uk/media/schools/management/documents/Case-4-Food-Promotion- to-Children.pdf>. Accessed on: 28 Feb. 2013.

MCKEE, Martin Trust me, I'm an expert' Why expert advisory groups must change, Editor in Chief. **European Journal Of Public Health**. v.9, n.3, 1999.

MEERMAN, J; CARISMA, B.; THOMPSON, B. **Global, regional and subregional trends in undernourishment and malnutrition.** June, 2012. Available at: <http://www.fao.org/fileadmin/user_upload/agn/pdf/SOFA_2013global.regional.subre gio nal.trends.pdf> Accessed: Dec. 9, 2013.

MINAYO, Cecilia. **The challenge of knowledge: qualitative research in health.** 9. revised and improved edition, Sâo Paulo: Hucitec. 2006.

MITCHELL, H. S. et al. **Nutrition.** 1.ed. Rio de Janeiro: Ed Interamericana Ltda, 1978.

MITCHELL Marc. An overview of public private partnerships in health. Boston: Harvard School of Public Health; 2008. Available at: <https://www.hsph.harvard.edu/ihsg/publications/pdf/PPP-final-MDM.pdf>. Accessed on: 02 Apr. 2014.

MOKHTAR, N: ELATI, J; CHABIR, R et al. Diet Culture and Obesity in Northern Africa. **Journal of Nutrition**, 131: 887S-892S, 2001. Available at: jn.nutrition.org. Accessed on: Aug. 20, 2009.

MONDINI L.; MONTEIRO C. Epidemiological relevance of malnutrition and obesity in different social classes: study methods and application to the Brazilian population. **Revista Brasileira de Epidemiologia,** v.2 n.1, p.28-39. 1998.

MONTEIRO, C.A et al. Endef and Pnsn: where is the physical growth of Brazilian children heading? **Cadernos de Saùde Pùblica**, Rio de Janeiro, v.9, supl.1, p.85-95, 1993.

. Nutrition and health: the issue is not food, nor nutrients, so much as processing. **Public Health Nutrition**, v.12, n.5, p.729-31. 2009.

. The big issue is ultra-processing. [Commentary] **World Nutrition,** v.1, n.6, 237259, nov. 2010. Available at: www.wphna.org. Accessed on: July 12, 2011.

;_CANNON, G.The Impact of Transnational "Big Food" Companies on the South: a view from Brazil. **PLoS Medicine**, v.9, n.7, jul. 2012. 2012. Available at:

<http://www.plosmedicine.org/article/fetchObject.action?uri=info%3Adoi%2F10.1371 %2 Fjournal.pmed.1001252&representation=PDF>. Accessed on: June 15, 2013.

CONDE, W.L.; DE CASTRO, I.R.R. A tendência cambiante da relação entre escolaridade e risco de obesidade no Brasil (1975-1997). **Cadernos de Saùde Pùblica**, v.19, sup.1, p.S67-S75. 2003.

MONTEIRO, C. A et al. Ultra-processed products are becoming dominant in the global food system. **Obesity Reviews,** v. 14, sup. 2, p.21-18. 2013. Available at:

<http://onlinelibrary.wiley.com/store/10.1111/obr.12107/asset/obr12107.pdf?v=1&t =i2l tdoo7&s=6129299271a6bb8948f5e1b76f8b18fb97fd5fcf>. Accessed on:17 Nov. 2014.

MOODIE, R. et al. Profits and pandemics:prevention of harmful effects of tobacco, alcohol and ultra-processed food and drink industries. **The Lancet**, v. 381, n. 9867, p.670 - 679, 2013. Available at: <http://www.thelancet.com/journals/lancet/article/PIIS0140-6736(12)62089-3/abstract>. Accessed on: 12 Dec. 2013.

MUST, Aviva. Morbidity and mortality associated with elevated body weight in children and adolescents. **American Journal Clinical Nutrition**, v.63, n.3, p.445S-447S, mar. 1996.

NARDOCCI, Adelaide Càssia. Social Risk Management. **Revista de Direito Sanitàrio**, v. 3, n.1, p.64-78, mar. 2002.

NESTLE, Marion. Food Marketing and Childhood Obesity: a matter of policy. **N Engl J Med,** v.354, n.24, p. 2527-2529, 2006. Available at: <www.nejm.org june 15>. Accessed on: March 31, 2014.

NEWELL D.G. et al. Food-borne diseases- the challenges of 20 years ago still persist while new ones continue to emerge. **International Journal of Food Microbiology**, v.30, n.139, suppl. 1, p.S3-15, may. 2010

NOBRE, M. R. et al. Prevalence of overweight, obesity and lifestyle habits associated with cardiovascular risk in elementary school students. **Revista da** Associaçâo **Médica Brasileira,** Sâo Paulo, v.52, n.2, p.118-124, 2006.

NILSON, E.A.F.; JAIME, P.C.; RESENDE, D.O. Initiatives developed in Brazil to reduce sodium content in processed foods. **Revista Panamericana Salud Publica**, v.32, n.4, p.287-92, 2012.

ORLANDI, Eni Puccinelli. **Discourse analysis: principles and procedures.** 9. ed. Campinas, SP: Pontes Editores, 2010.

OLIVEIRA, R. O.; ELIAS, P. E. M. Concepts of health regulation in Brazil. **Revista de Saùde Pùblica**, v.46, n.3, p.571-576. 2012.

OLIVEIRA-CAMPOS, M; RODRIGUES-NETO, JF; SILVEIRA, MF; NEVES, DMR; et al. Impact of risk factors for chronic non-communicable diseases on quality of life. **Ciência & Saùde Coletiva**, v.18, n.3, p.873-882, 2013.

PECI, Alketa. New regulatory framework for post-privatization Brazil: the role of regulatory agencies in question. State Reform and Governance Studies and Research Program. **Revista de Administraçào Pùblica**, Rio de Janeiro, v.33, n.4, p.121:35, jul/ago. 1999.

PÊCHEUX, Michel. **O Discurso: estrutura ou acontecimento**, 5th Edition, Campinas, SP: Pontes Editores, 2008.

PETERSON, A.; LUPTON, D. **The new public health: health and self in the age of risk.** London: SAGE Publication Ltda. 2000.

PETKANTCHIN, Valentin. **Nutrition" taxes: the costs of Denmark's fat tax. IEM's Economic Note ·may**, 2013. Available at:

<http://www.institutmolinari.org/IMG/pdf/note0513_en.pdf>. Accessed on: June 26, 2014.

PHILIPPI, Sônia Tucunduva. Food guide for the year 2000. In: DE ANGELIS, R. C. **Hidden hunger, physiological bases for reducing your risk through healthy eating**. Sâo Paulo: Editora Atheneu, chapter 9, 2000, p.160-176.

PHILLIPS, Lynne. Food and globalization. **Annual Review of Anthropology**, p.35:37-57. 2006.

PINGALI, P.; KHWAJA, Y. **Globalization of Indian Diets and the Transformation of Food Supply Systems . ESA Working Paper No. 04-05,** February 2004. Inaugural Keynote Address 17th Annual Conference Indian Society of Agricultural Marketing Hyderabad, February 5-7, 2004. Agricultural and Development Economics Division. The Food and Agriculture Organization of the United Nations. Available at: <http://ageconsearch.umn.edu/bitstream/23796/1/wp040005.pdf>. Accessed on: November 23, 2013.

PINHEIRO, A.R.O.; FREITAS, S.F.T.; CORSO, A.C.T. An epidemiological approach to obesity. **Revista de Nutriçào,** v.17, n.4, p.523-533, Oct./Dec. 2004.

PINTO, A. R. et al. Manual de normalização de trabalhos acadêmicos. 2. ed. rev. e atual.

Viçosa, MG: The Authors, 2011. Available at: <http://www.bbt.ufv.br/docs/ManualtrabalhosAcademicosLinks.pdf>. Accessed: March 15, 2013.

PONS, Silvia Carrasco. Theoretical and Methodological Starting Points for the Sociocultural Study of Food in a Context of Transformation. In: Canesqui, AM & Garcia, RWD (eds). **Anthropology and Nutrition: a possible dialog**. Rio de Janeiro: Editora Fiocruz, p.101-126. 2005.

POPKIN, Barry M. The nutrition transition and obesity in the developing world. Symposium: obesity in developing countries: biological and ecological factors. **The Journal of Nutrition,** v.131, n.3, p. 871S-873S, mar. 2001.

. The Shift in Stages of the Nutrition Transition in the Developing World Differs from Past Experiences!.**Malaysian Journal of Nutrition**, v. 8, n.1, p.109-124, 2002.

. Global nutrition dynamics: the world is shifting rapidly toward a diet linked with noncommunicable diseases. **American Journal of Clinical Nutrition,** n.84, p.289-98, 2006.

;_**GORDON-LARSEN**, P. The nutrition transition: worldwide obesity dynamics and their determinants. **International Journal of Obesity,** n.28 p.S2-S9, 2004.

PRADO JR. Caio. **Economic history of Brazil.** Sâo Paulo: Editora Brasiliense, 36th edition, 1988.

PRENTICE, Andrew M. The emerging epidemic of obesity in developing countries.

International Journal of Epidemiology, v.35, p.93-99, 2005.

PUSKA, Pekka. Successful strategies to influence national diets: the Finnish experience. **Zdrav Varv**, v.43, p.191-196, 2004.

QUEIROZ, L.G.; GIOVANELLA, L. Regional health agenda in Mercosur: architecture and themes. **Revista Panamericana de Salud Publica**, v.30, n.2, p.182-188, 2011.

RAYNER, G; HAWKES, C; LANG, T & BELLO, W. Trade liberalization and diet transition: a public health response. **Health Promotion International**, v.21, n.S1, p.67-74, 2007.

Available at: <http://heapro.oxfordjournals.org>. Accessed on: 16 Nov. 2013.

RECINE, E.; MORTOZA, A. S. **Consenso sobre habilidades e competências do nutricionista no âmbito da saùde coletiva**, Brasilia: Observatório de Politicas de Segurança e Nutriçâo, 2013. Available at:

<http://www.crn2.org.br/download/12_12_2013_17_32_43_consenso.pdf>. Accessed on: June 15, 2014.

REGMI, A & GEHLHAR, M. Processed Food Trade Pressured by Evolving Global Supply Chains. Economic Research SERVICE/USDA. **Amber Waves** 12, v.3, n.1. feb. 2005.

Available at: <www.ers.usda.gov/amberwaves>. Accessed on: 28 nov.2013.

RIBEIRO, J.M.; COSTA, N.R.; SILVA, P.L.B. Politica de Saùde no Brasil e estratégias regulatórias em ambiente de mudanças tecnológicas, Interface - **Comunicaçâo, Saùde, Educaçâo**, v.4, n.6, p. 61-84, 2000.

ROBERTSON, Aileen. Social inequalities and the burden of food-related ill-health. **Public Health Nutrition**, v.4, n.6, p.1371-1373, 2001.

ROBINSON, T.N. et al. Effects of fast food branding on young children's taste preferences. **Archives of Pediatrics & Adolescent Medicine**, v.161, n.8, p.792-797, 2007.

RODRIGUES, E.M.; TADDEI, J.A.A.C.; SIGULEM, D.M. Overweight and obesity among mothers of malnourished children - Brazil - PNSN - 1989. **Sâo Paulo Medical Journal,** v. 116, n.4, p.1766-1773, jul. 1998.

RONQUE, E. R. et al. Prevalence of overweight and obesity in schoolchildren of high socioeconomic status in Londrina, Paranà, Brazil. **Revista de Nutriçâo**, Campinas, v.18, n.6, p.709-717, nov./dez. 2005.

ROSAS, Erick Jenner. The enemies of health reform mobilize. **Saùde em Debate.** v.22, p.13-18, Oct. 1988.

SANTOS, Andréia Mendes. **Consumer Society: children and advertising, a relationship that gives weight.** Porto Alegre: EDIPUCRS, 2009.

SANTOS, Boaventura de Sousa. The critique of neoliberal governance: The World Social Forum as politics and subaltern cosmopolitan legality. Revista Critica de Ciências Sociais, v.72, p.7-44, Oct. 2005.

SAVE THE CHILDREN. A life free from hunger: tackling child malnutrition. London: Save The Children, 2012. Available at:

<http://www.savethechildren.org.uk/sites/default/files/images/A_Life_Free_From_Hu nge r.pdf">. Accessed on: September 18, 2013.

SCALLAN, Elaine. Activities, Achievements, and Lessons Learned during the First 10 Years of the Foodborne Diseases Active Surveillance Network: 1996-2005. **Clinical Infectious Diseases**, n.44, n.7, p.18-25. 2007.

SCHAFER, K.S.; KEGLEY, S.E. Persistent toxic chemicals in the US food supply. Journal of Epidemiology and Community Health, v.56, p.813-817. 2002.

SCHMIDT, M.I. et al. Chronic non-communicable diseases in Brazil: burden and current challenges. Published online May 9, 2011. Available at: <http://www.sbh.org.br/pdf/lancet_collection.pdf>. Accessed on: August 16, 2013.

SEIPEL, Michael M. O. Social Consequences of Malnutrition. **Social Work** , v.44, n.5, p.416425, sep.1999.

SINGER, P. Evoluçâo da Economia Brasileira: 1955-1975. **Estudos CEBRAP,** Sâo Paulo, n. 17, p.61-83, jul-set, 1976. Available at:

<www.cebrap.org.br/v2/files/upload/biblioteca_virtual/evolucao_da_economia_brasile ira. pdf>. Accessed on: July 22, 2014.

SOUTO, Ana Cristina. **Health and Politics: Health Surveillance in Brazil, 1976-1994**. Sâo

Paulo: Sobravime, 2004. 227p.

SKLAIR, Leslie. Democracy and the Transnational Capitalist Class. **ANNALS, AAPSS**, n.581, p.144-157, may. 2002,

STUCKLER, D; NESTLE, M. Big food, food systems, and global health. **PLoS Medicine,** v.9, n.6, e1001242, jun. 2012. Available at:

<http://www.plosmedicine.org/article/fetchObiect.action?uri=info%3Adoi%2F10.1371 %2 Fjournal.pmed.1001242&representation=PDF>. Accessed on September 15, 2013.

SWINBURN, B.A. et al. Diet, nutrition and the prevention of excess weight gain and obesity.

Public Health Nutrition, v.7, n.1A, p.123-146, 2004.

TANAKA, K.; NAKANISHI, T. Obesity as a risk factor for various diseases: necessity of lifestyle changes for healthy aging. **Applied Human Science**, v.15, n.4, p.139-148, 1996.

TAORMINA, PJ; BEUCHAT, L.R.; SLUTSKER, L. Infections Associated with Eating Seed

Sprouts: **An International Concern. Emerging Infectious Diseases.** v. 5, n. 5, , p.626-634, sep./oct. 1999.

TAUXE, Robert V. International investigation of outbreaks of foodborne disease: Public health responds to the globalization of food. **British Medical Journal**, v. 313, n. 2, p.10931094, nov.1996.

. Emerging foodborne diseases: an evolving public health challenge. **Emerging infectious diseases.** v.3, n.4, p.425-434, oct./dec.1997.

TERRES, N.G. et al. Prevalence and factors associated with overweight and obesity in adolescents. Prevalence and factors associated with overweight and obesity in adolescents. **Revista Saùde Pùblica**, v.40, n.4, p.627-633, aug. 2006.

THOMPSON, John. B **Ideology and modern culture: critical social theory in the age of the mass media**. 8. ed. Petrópolis, RJ: Vozes, 2009.

THOW, A.M.; HAWKES, C. The implications of trade liberalization for diet and health: a case study from Central America. **Globalization and Health** 2009. Available at: <http://www.globalizationandhealth.com/content/5/1/5>. Accessed on: 15 Nov. 2012.

TORUN B; CHEW F. Energy-protein malnutrition. In: SHILS, O.; SHIKE, R. (eds). **Treatise on modern nutrition in health and disease.** Barueri/SP: Ed. Manole Ltda, 1029-1056, 2003.

TULLAO, Tereso S. **The Impact of Economic Globalization on Noncommunicable Diseases: Opportunities and Threats**. In: WHO. Globalization, diets and noncommunicable diseases. Switzerland:WHO Library Cataloguing-in-Publication Data. 2002.

UNITED KINDOWN. Food Standards Agency. **Front-of-pack traffic light signpost labeling**. Technical guidance. n. 2, November, 2007. Available at: <http://multimedia.food.gov.uk/multimedia/pdfs/frontofpackguidance2.pdf.> Accessed on: June 24, 14.

UNITED NATIONS. **International Covenant on Economic, Social and Cultural Rights**. Adopted and opened for signature, ratification and accession by General Assembly resolution 2200A (XXI) of December 16, 1966. Available at: <http://www.ohchr.org/EN/ProfessionalInterest/Pages/cescr.aspx>. Accessed on Aug. 10, 2014.

. **World Population Prospects: The 2012 Revision.** Available at: http://esa.un.org/unpd/wpp/Excel-Data/population.htm. Accessed on: November 29, 2013.

. **Political Declaration of the High-level Meeting of the General Assembly on the Prevention and Control of Non-communicable Diseases** Resolution adopted by the General Assembly. 24 jan. 2012. Available at:

<http://www.who.int/nmh/events/un_ncd_summit2011/political_declaration_en.pdf>. Accessed on: June 23, 2014

UUSITALLO, U.; PIETINEN, P.; PEKKA, P. Dietary transition in developing countries: challenges for chronic disease prevention. In: WORLD HEALTH ORGANIZATION.

Globalization diets and noncommunicable diseases. Switzerland:WHO Library, p.1-25, 2002.

VALENTE, Flàvio Luiz Shieck. Hunger, malnutrition and citizenship: social inclusion and human rights. Saùde e Sociedade v.12, n.1, p.51-60, jan-jun. 2003.

VASCONCELOS, V.L.; SILVA, G.A.P. Prevalência de sobrepeso e obesidade em adolescentes masculinos, no Nordeste do Brasil, 1980 a 2000. **Cadernos Saùde Pùblica** , v.19, n.5, p.1445-1451, set-out. 2003.

VEPA, Swarna Sadasivan. Impact of globalization on the food consumption of urban India. In: Globalization of food systems in developing countries: impact on food security and nutrition FAO. **Food Nutrition Paper 83,** 2004, Reprinted, p. 215-330, 2006.

VISSCHER, T.L.S.; SEIDELL, J.C. The public health impact of obesity. **Annual Review Public Health**, v.22, p.355-375, 2001.

WEBER, R. et al. Dioxin- and POP-contaminated sites-contemporary and future relevance and challenges: Overview on background, aims and scope of the series. **Environmental Science and Pollution Research**, v.15, p.363-393, 2008.

WEISS, A.R.; MCMICHAEL, A.J. Social and environmental risk factors in the emergence of infectious diseases. **Nature Medicine Supplement,** v. 10, n. 12, p. S70-S76, dec. 2004.

WILLET, Walter. **Nutritional epidemiology.** New York: Oxford University, 1990.

WORLD HEALTH ORGANIZATION. **The role of food safety**. Report of Joint FAO/WHO Expert Committee on Food Safety. Geneve, Switzerland:WHO. 1984. (WHO Technical Report series n. 705).

. **Diet, nutrition and the prevention of chronic diseases. Report of a WHO study group.** Geneve, Switzerland: WHO Library Cataloguing in Publication Data, 1990 (World Health Organization technical report series; 797).

. **The world health report 1998 Life in the 21st century: a vision for all.**

Geneve, Switzerland: WHO Library Cataloguing in Publication Data. 1998. Accessed on: 7/12/2013. Available at: http://www.who.int/whr/1998/en/whr98_en.pdf

. **Report WHO Consultation on Diagnostic Procedures for Transmissible Spongiform Encephalopathies: Need for Reference Reagents and Reference Panels.**

Geneva, Switzerland 22-23 March 1999. World Health Organization Blood Safety and Clinical Technology June 1999.

. **Turning the tide of malnutrition: respond to the challenge of 21st century.**

2000 WHO/NHD/00.7. Available at: < http://whqlibdoc.who.int/hq/2000/WHO NHD 00.7.pdf>. Accessed on: Aug. 17, 2013.

. **Reducing Risks, Promoting Healthy Life**. The world health report 2002. Switzerland: WHO Library Cataloguing in Publication Data, 2002a.

. **Global surveillance of foodborne disease: developing a strategy and its interaction with risk analysis**. Geneve, Switzerland, November 26-29, 2001. Report of WHO Consultation, 2002b.

. **The present state of foodborne disease in OECD countries.** Geneve:WHO Document Production Service, 2003a. Available at:

<http://www.who.int/foodsafety/publications/foodborne disease/oecd fbd.pdf>. Accessed on: Aug. 12, 2013.

. Joint WHO/FAO Expert Consultation on Diet, Nutrition and the Prevention of Chronic Diseases (2002 : Geneva, Switzerland) **Diet, nutrition and the prevention of chronic diseases: report of a joint WHO/FAO expert consultation**, Geneva, 28 January - 1 February 2002. 2003b. (WHO technical report series ; 916).

. **Global Health: today's challenges**. Chapter one. p.1-22, 2003c. Available at <http://www.who.int/whr/2003/en/Chapter1-en.pdf?ua=1>. Accessed on: 19 Nov. 2014.

. **Obesity: preventing and managing the global epidemic**; Report of a WHO consultation. Geneve, Switzerland: WHO Library Cataloguing in Publication Data (World Health Organization technical report series; 894), 2000. Reprinted 2004a.

. **Global Strategy on Diet, Physical Activity and Health.** Fifty Seventh World Health Assembly WHA57.17. Agenda item 12.6. 22 may France, WHO, 2004b.

. **Preventing chronic diseases: a vital investment**. WHO global report. Switzerland: WHO Library Cataloguing-in-Publication Data. 2005.

. **The challenge of obesity in the WHO European Region and the strategies for response**. European Ministerial Conference on Counteracting Obesity. Instanbul, Turkey, November 15-17, 2006.

. **The global burden of foodborne disease: taking stock and charting the way forward**. WHO Consultation to Develop a Strategy to Estimate the Global Burden of Foodborne Diseases. Geneva, 25-27 september. 2006. Geneva: WHO Press; 2007. Available: <http://www.who.int/foodsafety/publications/foodborne_disease/burden_sept06/en. 2007.>. Accessed on: August 12, 2013.

. **Initiative to estimate the global burden of foodborne diseases**. A summary document. 2008. Available at: <http://www.who.int/foodsafety/foodborne disease/Summary Doc.pdf?ua=1>. Accessed on: May 08, 2012.

. **Infant and young child nutrition.** Sixty-third World Health Assembly A63/9. Provisional agenda item 11.6 1 april 2010, Report by the Secretariat. Available at: <http://apps.who.int/gb/ebwha/pdf_files/WHA63/A63_9-en.pdf>. Accessed on: Feb. 25, 2012.

. **World health statistics 2011**. Switzerland:WHO Library Cataloguing-in-Publication Data. Available at: <http://www.who.int/gho/publications/world_health_statistics/EN_WHS2011_Full.pdf > Accessed on: 25 Feb. 2012.

. **Global nutrition policy review: what does it take to scale up nutrition action?** Geneva, Switzerland:WHO Library Cataloguing-in-Publication Data. 2013a. Disponivel em: http://apps.who.int/iris/bitstream/10665/84408/1/9789241505529 eng.pdf?ua=1. Accessed on: Feb. 14, 2014.

. **Draft comprehensive global monitoring framework and targets for the prevention and control of noncommunicable diseases**. Report by the Director-General. Sixty-Sixth World Health Assembly A66/8. Provisional agenda item 13.1 15 March 2013b. Accessed on: July 3, 2014.

. Dioxins and their effects on human health. **Fact sheet N°225.** Updated June 2014. Available at: http://www.who.int/mediacentre/factsheets/fs225/en/>. Accessed on: 18 Nov. 2014.

WORLD TRADE ORGANIZATION. **World Trade Report 2008**. Trading in a globalizing world. Available:

<http://www.wto.org/english/res_e/booksp_e/anrep_e/world_tradea_report08_e.pdf> Accessed on: 13 Nov. 2013

. **Understanding The WTO: The Organization. Members and Observers.** Home page. 2013a. Available at: http://www.wto.org/english/thewto_e/whatis_e/tif_e/org6_e.htm. Accessed on: 13 Nov. 2013.

. **WTO II Merchandising Trade**. International Trade Statistics 2013. 2013b Available at: www.wto.org/statistics. Accessed on: 13 Nov. 2013.

. **List of tables II. Merchandise trade by product.** World Trade

Organization International Trade Statistics 2013c. Available at: www.wto.org/statistics. Accessed on: 13 Nov. 2013.

ZIMMERMAN, F.J.; BELL, J.F. Associations of Television Content Type and Obesity in Children. **American Journal of Public Health,** v.100, n. 2, p. 334-340, feb. 2010.

ANNEXES

ANNEX I. Informed Consent Form.

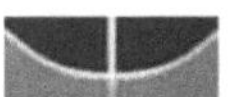

UNIVERSITY OF BRASILIA

FACULTY OF HEALTH SCIENCES

NUTRITION DEPARTMENT

POSTGRADUATE PROGRAM IN HUMAN NUTRITION

free and clear consent form

Dear,

You are being invited to take part in the research project "Emerging food risks: the Brazilian regulatory strategy from the perspective of social actors". The main objective of this research is to characterize how different social actors understand emerging food risks that affect public health. The information obtained will be used exclusively for this research and will be published in a consolidated form (without exposing the names of the participants), in the form of a doctoral thesis and a scientific article. No professional will have their data disclosed individually, and anonymity and the preservation of the information provided will be guaranteed. We would also like to inform you that there is no direct and/or individual benefit for the participant and that no procedure will be carried out that will cause them any discomfort, risk to their health and/or expense of any kind.

The survey consists of an interview lasting approximately one hour. Your participation is fundamental to the research. Thank you in advance for your contribution.

This research corresponds to a project for the preparation of the main researcher's doctoral thesis, a requirement of the Postgraduate Program in Human Nutrition. It aims to analyze public food regulation policies aimed at controlling emerging food risks.

You will have access, at any time, to information about the procedures, risks and benefits related to the research, including to resolve any doubts. In addition, you will be free to withdraw your consent at any time and to stop taking part in the study, without this causing any harm, as well as to refuse to answer any questions that may cause you embarrassment.

Contact details of the researcher responsible: Student Ana Virginia de Almeida Figueiredo,

Observatory of Food and Nutrition Policies, Faculty of Sciences (61) 3034-6526 End: SQN 216, Bloco "D" , apt 209, Asa Norte, (61) 9964-9305 Research Ethics Committee, Faculty of Health Sciences, Darcy Ribeiro Campus, Nutrition Center, room 9, Asa Norte, University of Brasilia, (61) 9964-9305 and (61) 3307-2508.

RESEARCH SUBJECT IDENTIFICATION DATA

1. Name:	
2. Body (federal/district):	
3. Function:	4. Sex: M ( ) F ( )
5. Contact telephone number: ( )	
6. Manager ( ) Health Counselor ( ) Health Professional ( )SUS user ( )	

Brasilia, 20

Signature of Research Subject (stamp or legible name)

Researcher's signature

(stamp or legible name)

NOTE: The sheets will be initialed by the research subject and the researcher in charge.

ANNEX II. Interview script.

UNIVERSITY OF BRASÍLIA

FACULTY OF HEALTH SCIENCES

NUTRITION DEPARTMENT

POSTGRADUATE PROGRAM IN HUMAN NUTRITION

PHD IN NUTRITION

INTERVIEWEE PROFILE

Id:

Academic background: ____

Institution: ____

Position held: ____

Length of experience in the institution: ____________________

---

1. What activities do you carry out related to food or food-related problems?

2. How long have you been doing this job?

3. In your opinion, what is the relationship between excess weight and food?

A) What measures can you highlight to reduce the impact of food on excess weight?

B) In your opinion, how should institutions organize themselves to control excess weight?

C) What specific role does your organization/institution play in this context?

D) What would be the responsibilities of the government and the other sectors involved in the process of regulating the emerging risks of overweight foods?

E) What is your assessment of the strategy of expanding food regulation activities by the public authorities in order to curb excess weight?

F) How can health surveillance with a focus on food act to interfere with excess weight?

G) What facilities and difficulties exist for intervening on the risks of food related to excess weight?

H) In your opinion, has the process of economic globalization, specifically in the field of food, interfered with the quality of food and the health of the population?

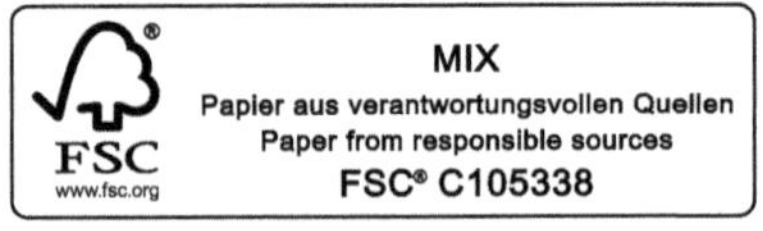

Printed by Books on Demand GmbH, Norderstedt / Germany